101 BEAUTY TIPS

101 BEAUTY TIPS

Jane Cunningham

q RA778.C86 2007
Cunningham, Jane, 1965–
101 beauty tips
Buffalo, N.Y. : Firefly
Books, 2007.

FIREFLY BOOKS

A FIREFLY BOOK

Published by Firefly Books Ltd. 2007

First printing

Publisher Cataloging-in-Publication Data (U.S.)

Cunningham, Jane.
   101 Beauty Tips / Jane Cunningham.
[192] p. : col. photos. ; cm.
Includes index.

Summary: Includes hair and skin care, makeup, healthy diet, physical fitness and stress management.

ISBN-13: 978-1-55407-245-3 (pbk.)

ISBN-10: 1-55407-245-X (pbk.)

1. Beauty, Personal. 2. Women—Health and hygiene. I. Title.

646.7042 dc22   RA778.A2.C866 2007

Library and Archives Canada Cataloguing in Publication

Cunningham, Jane, 1965-
   101 beauty tips / Jane Cunningham.

Includes index.
ISBN-13: 978-1-55407-245-3
ISBN-10: 1-55407-245-X

1. Beauty, Personal. 2. Health. I. Title. II. Title: One hundred and one beauty tips. III. Title: One hundred one beauty tips.

RA778.C85 2007   646.7'2   C2006-904596-8

Published in the United States by
Firefly Books (U.S.) Inc.
P.O. Box 1338, Ellicott Station
Buffalo, New York 14205

Published in Canada by
Firefly Books Ltd.
66 Leek Crescent
Richmond Hill, Ontario L4B 1H1

Manufactured in Singapore by Pica Digital (Pte) Ltd
Printed in Singapore by Star Standard Industries (Pte) Ltd

It is always sensible to consult your doctor before changing your diet or starting a new exercise regime, but it is essential to do so if you suffer from any medical condition or are taking medication of any kind. If you are concerned about any symptoms that develop after changing your diet or your exercise regime, consult your doctor immediately. Information is given without any guarantees on the part of the author and Publisher, and they cannot be held responsible for the contents of this book.

CONTENTS

Introduction

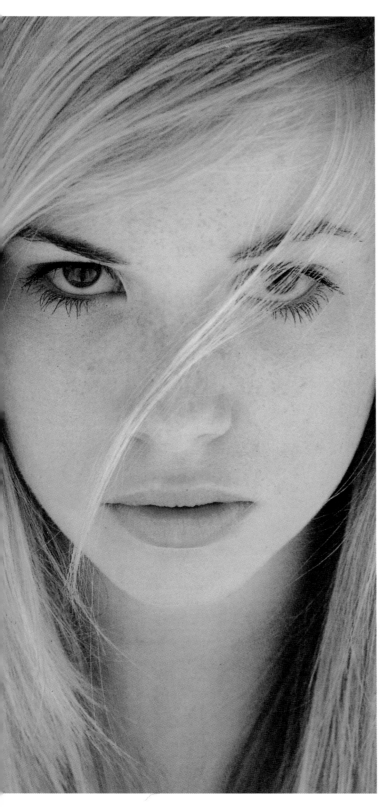

The 21st century beauty industry has launched a whole new stratosphere of high-tech skin care and treatments, all promising to rejuvenate, banish wrinkles and give you younger-looking skin. Some of it works, to a degree, and some of it doesn't. But what will really give your well-being and skin the edge is using a mind and body approach to stay at your most healthy and relaxed. There is no wonder cream in the world that will cure you of tiredness, stress or obesity, but incorporating a few of our valuable tips into your life really could make the difference to both how you look and how you feel. We don't concentrate on advanced cosmeceuticals, but more on what nature, what you eat and good health routines can do in terms of your physical appearance, both for skin and body.

The makeup and skin care section is designed to give you a good basic knowledge of what products are actually for, and the best way to use them. Makeup is an important part of almost every woman's life, and knowing how to use it properly and to make the most of your looks is a big advantage and a confidence booster.

Relaxation is fundamental to how we look; beautiful, clear and healthy skin is a reflection of how you feel inside. Getting good-quality sleep and regular moments of tranquility in your life will allow you to shine on the inside and glow on the outside.

Perhaps most important is our section on exercise. We now know that it is so important to incorporate exercise into your life not only for longevity and health, but for a vitality that will show in your eyes, face and body. There is no better way to raise self-esteem and throw off clouds of anxiety than to exercise. Work hard to find a regime that you like, and watch the pounds disappear, see your body change to a shape that you'll love, and wait for the years to fall off your face.

However you choose to look after your skin, you will read that the most important thing you can do right now is to wear a sunscreen with an appropriate SPF (sun protection factor) for your skin type. Skin that has been overexposed to the sun not only runs the risk of severe damage, but looks and acts older than it is. It is never too soon to start using sunscreen to prevent sun damage, and thankfully, never too late to gain some benefits.

You will also find that what you eat and drink is a key player in the way that you look and feel. Fresh looks come from fresh food and water; smooth, soft and clear skin is a happy byproduct of keeping your hydration levels up and eating healthfully. But we never say never! When it comes to eating and drinking, use moderation not starvation as your watchword, and you will reap the long-term beauty benefits over and over with our real solutions for real women.

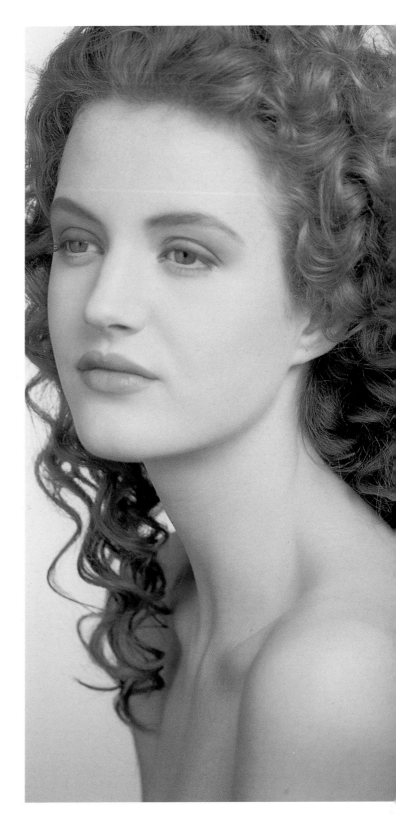

chapter one
HEALTHY HAIR

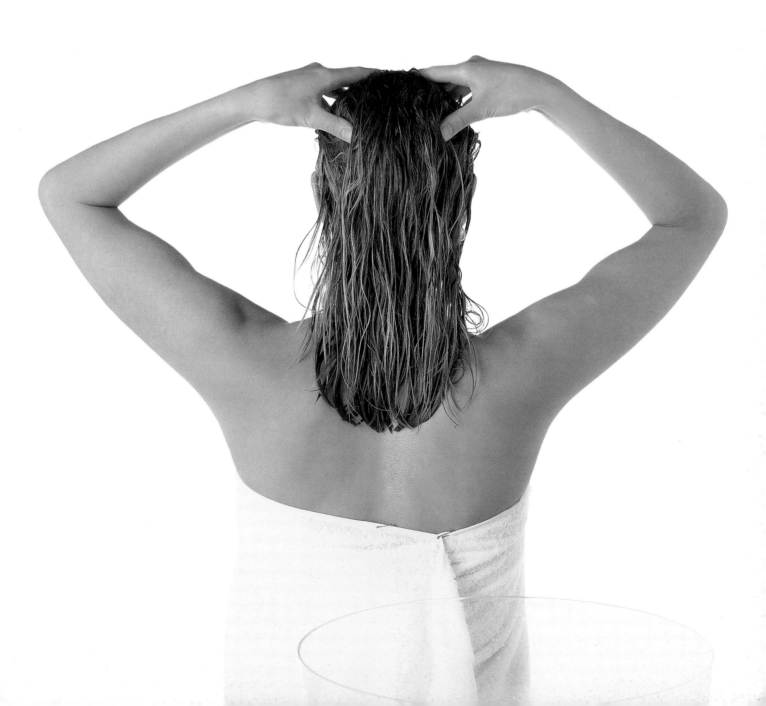

Tip 1: *Washing Your Hair*

Your hair is a valuable natural fiber and to get it looking its best you should treat it with as much care as you would silk or wool. Fortunately, hair is very resilient. An average single hair can be stretched by 20 to 30 percent its normal length — a force that would snap most textile fabrics. Wet hair needs less force to stretch it and is more vulnerable to damage. If your hair is in poor condition because of neglect, or if it has been subjected to harsh treatment, all is not lost. With care and attention you should be able to restore its bounce and glossy sheen.

Your hair type is inherited, but learning to make the most of what you have can make a difference to the look, feel and texture of your crowning glory. There are plenty of myths surrounding the seemingly simple process of hair washing. Does washing your hair every day make it greasy? Do you need to spend a fortune on shampoo? Does a rinse of freezing water make your hair shine? The answer to all is no, but there are a few hard and fast rules that will benefit both your hair and scalp.

Most hair washing products advise that two washes are essential; this simply isn't true. Unless your hair is unusually dirty, normal hair reacts and cleans perfectly well with one good wash, using roughly a dollar-coin-sized amount of shampoo in the palm of your hand. Bear in mind, though, that if you live in a hard-water area, you may need more. It's a good idea to rub your hands together to distribute the shampoo before applying it to your hair. That way, it is less likely that you will end up with one big lump on the top of your head that then has to be worked down through the hair.

Trichologists (hair specialists) advise clients with thinning or troublesome hair to massage their scalp every time they shampoo, as this stimulates the scalp, increasing blood flow. Hair is made from the protein keratin, and is fed by blood vessels at the roots, so increasing the flow gives hair a nutrient boost. A scalp massage is easily done by placing fingers spread apart over your head, and gently kneading the scalp for two minutes.

No matter what your hair type, and no matter what shampoo you choose, the key to glossy, clean locks is to rinse, rinse and rinse again. Even when you think that every last drop of shampoo is out, give yourself at least another couple of minutes under the shower to get rid of the very last remnants. Smooth your hair under the water flow over and over again; ruffling it disturbs the hair shafts making it less likely to be sleek.

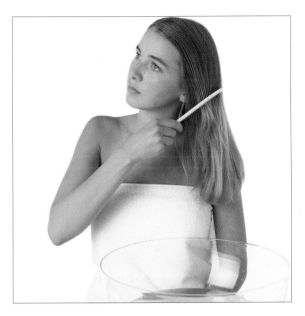

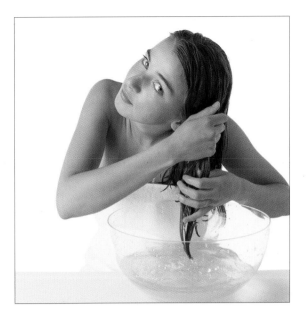

1. To avoid tangles while shampooing, run a wide-toothed comb through your dry hair. Remove any knots from the ends, then gradually work your way up toward the roots. Once you have rid the hair of tangles, brush it to help remove any dust, dirt and dead skin cells. Brushing also increases the blood circulation of the scalp, helping to rejuvenate hair, aid new growth and redistribute the natural oils.

2. Next, presoak your hair (so that you need less shampoo). Apply warm water and gently draw your fingers through the hair as the water flows through it. Tug gently at the hair near to the scalp to improve circulation.

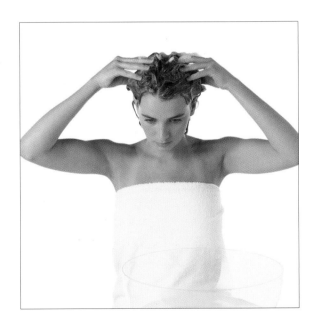

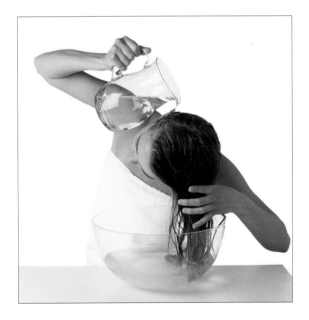

3. Pour a little shampoo into the palm of one hand and rub your hands together. Smooth your hands over your head to apply the shampoo, moving your hands from the root of your hair down toward the ends. Carefully massage the scalp with your fingertips for a couple of minutes. Every few seconds, run your fingers through your hair from top to bottom to make sure there are no tangles.

4. The final, all-important stage is rinsing. This is vital for healthy, shiny hair. The reason many people have dull hair is that it is covered with a thin film of shampoo residue. Even if you think your hair is sufficiently rinsed, do it just one more time. Finish with a final rinse of cold water to refresh and invigorate the scalp, then condition your hair. There is no need to shampoo more than once, unless there is a lot of dirt or sand in your hair.

Tip 2: *After Shampooing*

Shampooing causes the hair cuticles (the outer hair cells) to interlock and can lead to tangles. Conditioning the hair smooths these cells, so that you can comb your hair more easily. A conditioner also gives the hair extra shine. You should always apply conditioner after swimming, because chlorine dries out the hair.

Regardless of type, most hair benefits from a conditioning rinse, leaving hair shafts smoothed and flat. Not only does this mean that combing and brushing are easier, but styling is more manageable too. There are many different sorts of conditioners available, with differing degrees of effectiveness, but they all act to coat the hair for a sleeker result. A cost-effective way to choose what is right for your hair is to buy trial sizes, available at drug stores, or to seek expert advice from your hairdresser.

Long, thick hair will need more conditioner than a short bob, for example, so when pouring the conditioner into your hands, take account of how much hair you actually have! Once again, a dollar-coin-sized amount will be fine for short hair; double it for longer locks. Putting the palms of your hands together, coat your hair with conditioner, starting at mid-length, and working down to the ends rather than on top. The hair lower down is likely to be less well conditioned, so save the last drops for the top of your head.

Smooth the conditioner through your hair, giving yourself a short scalp massage at the same time. Leave the conditioner in for a few moments – modern conditioners work quickly – and begin to rinse.

One of the reasons that hair always feels so wonderful after a trip to the hairdresser is that they are adept at getting rid of any excess product buildup. So, once again, rinsing is the key. Conditioners, by their very nature, are more time consuming to get out than shampoos, so pay careful attention to ensuring you have rinsed enough. Many people make the mistake of not rinsing their hair thoroughly after conditioning. However, it is essential to remove all traces of conditioner if your hair is to remain healthy, shiny and full of body.

Once your hair is completely clean, wrap it in a warm, fresh towel. Don't be tempted to scrub away at your towel-wrapped hair in the hopes of drying it. While the action will remove excess water, it will also undo all your efforts toward smooth, tangle-free hair. Instead, gently tug your hair with the towel, moving to dryer parts of your towel as you gradually squeeze out the water. Using a wide-toothed comb to brush through is essential – wet hair is much more fragile, and any excessive tugging can lead to breakage or damage.

The active ingredients used in commercial products are known as "cationic surfactants" – chemicals that are attracted to dry and damaged hair. However, they do little more than temporarily coat the hair. Conditioners made from natural ingredients tend to be more compatible with the composition of the hair, leaving it smoother and more manageable,

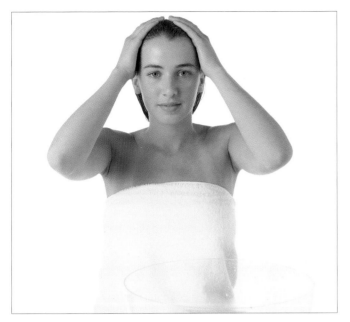

1. Pour a small amount of conditioner into the palm of your hand and rub your hands together. Run your hands over your hair, starting about 3–4 inches (8–10 cm) down from your scalp and working right to the ends. Never rub conditioner into your scalp or apply it to the hair near the scalp, since it could become greasy.

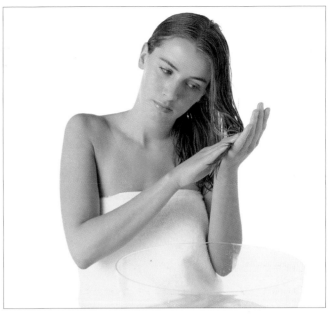

2. If you have long hair that is dry and damaged at the ends, apply a little extra conditioner to this area. Leave the conditioner on your hair for the length of time recommended on the bottle by the manufacturer; most commercially produced conditioners work virtually instantaneously.

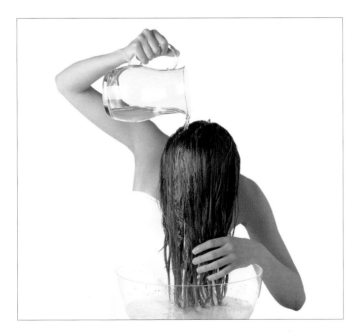

3. Rinse, rinse and rinse again; leaving a residue of conditioner on the hair will make it dull and limp. Finish with a cold-water rinse.

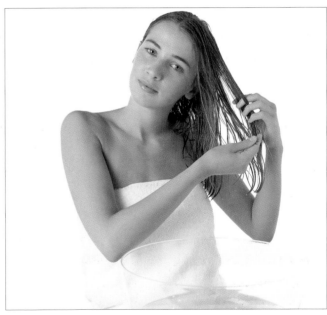

4. Wrap your hair in a thick cotton towel and press against the hair with your hands to absorb the excess moisture. Use a wide-toothed comb or your fingers to remove any tangles, starting at the ends of the hair.

Tip 3: *Diet Tips for Hair*

Just as with any part of your body, your hair will suffer if you do not eat the right foods. Although it is a cliché, you really are what you eat. Poor nutrition will leave hair feeling brittle and undernourished. A healthy diet will help your hair to stay strong and glossy.

Essential Fatty Acids

Salmon, mackerel, tuna and other oily fish are high in omega-3 fatty acids, which play an important role in strengthening skin, nails and hair. Other good sources include nuts – especially walnuts and almonds – and flaxseed oil.

Folic Acid & B Vitamins

In particular, vitamins B6 and B12 are thought to be of importance to the condition of your hair. Luckily, they are key players in a normal healthy diet, being found in fresh fruit and vegetables. Folic acid is found in beneficial quantities in whole-grain and fortified grain products, such as bread, and bananas, spinach and potatoes. As vegetarians and vegans can suffer from deficiencies in the major sources of vitamin B12, which is found in meat, poultry and dairy products, you may wish to consult a nutritionist about supplements.

Protein

Eating fish, chicken, lean meat, eggs and soy products are critical for protein intake, which has a direct effect on the health of your hair.

Trace Minerals

If you are unsure whether your diet is rich in trace minerals, such as magnesium and zinc, you may wish to consider a daily mineral supplement. Severe deficiencies in magnesium and zinc can lead to coarse, dry and brittle hair. If your hair doesn't suffer from these conditions, you probably have an adequately mineral-rich diet.

Tip 4: *Drying Hair*

If your hair could talk, it would ask you never to blow-dry it! However, letting hair dry naturally is usually not a practical option, and doesn't get the best-looking result for your hair. But, the more you blow-dry, the worse the condition of your hair will become. However, there are several ways to protect your hair from the worst effects of too much hot blow-drying.

When you have time, keep you dryer on its coolest setting. Even though it will take longer to dry your hair, those extra few minutes could be vital to the condition of your locks. Excessive heat is a major cause of hair dryness as it leaches away natural oils.

Invest in a heat protection spray, available at the drug store. These chemical products stop hair from drying out, and prevent heat-related damage, such as split ends and frizz.

Let your hair dry naturally as often as you can.

Whatever method you choose for drying hair, you should first comb it through. Start at the tip, easing the tangles gently out, and work back along the hair shaft. If you start at the scalp, you'll only create fiercer tangles lower down. Take your time and don't tug. Carelessness will damage your hair. Use a comb when the hair is wet, and you can switch to a brush once your hair is drier.

If you do not have time to let your hair dry naturally, ensure that you use your dryer on its coolest setting, as excessive heat can damage your hair.

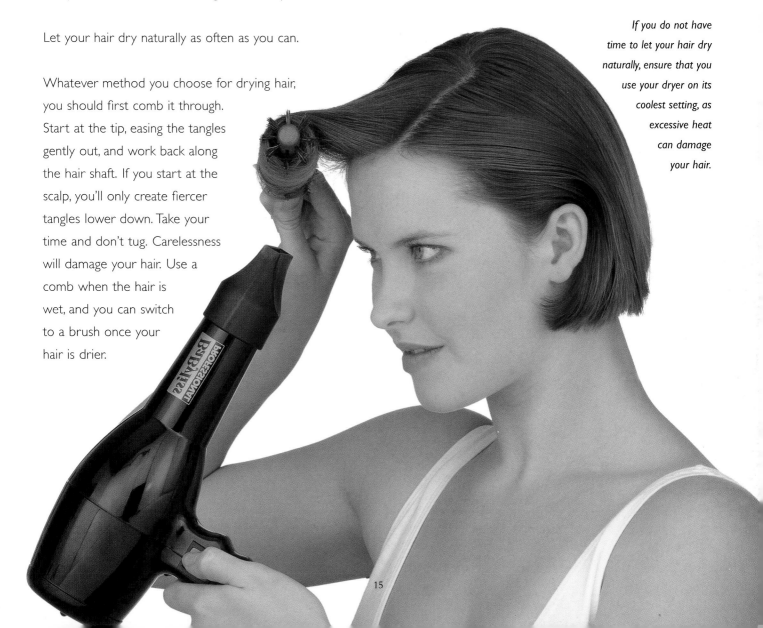

Tip 5: *Brushing Hair*

Using the correct brush for your hair type can make the difference between lackluster locks and shiny, vibrant hair. Although natural bristle brushes are thought to be best, soft nylon bristles won't "grab" and tear at hair, making them a good, and cheaper, alternative.

When brushing your hair, no matter what your hair type is, always proceed gently, and never be tempted to tug or rip. If you find that there are knots or snags in your hair, use a detangling spray (available at pharmacies) or a small amount of silicone based serum. This will smooth and soften the hair making it much easier to gently comb out a tangle.

Hair brushing stimulates the blood circulation to the scalp, helping your hair benefit from extra nutrients, and also evenly distributes natural oils, so spending time gently brushing can leave your hair in better condition. Those with hair prone to tangles may find that brushing the hair before washing and conditioning can help reduce knots, and brushing before bedtime can do the same.

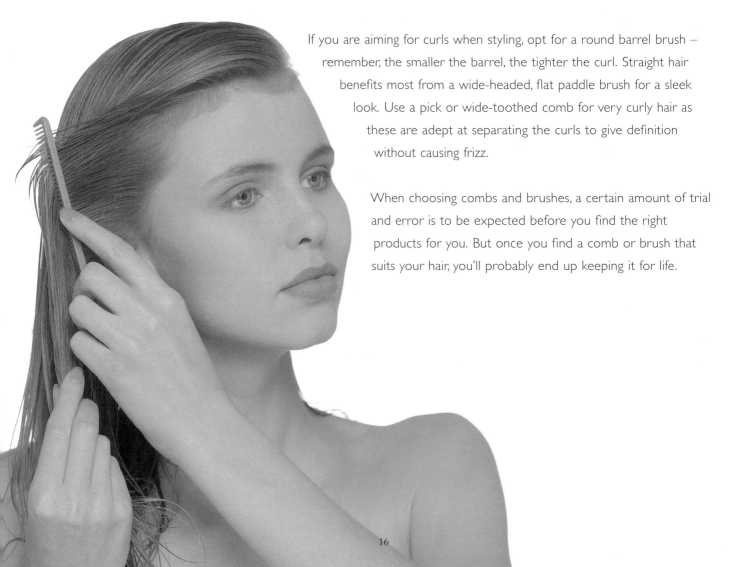

If you are aiming for curls when styling, opt for a round barrel brush – remember, the smaller the barrel, the tighter the curl. Straight hair benefits most from a wide-headed, flat paddle brush for a sleek look. Use a pick or wide-toothed comb for very curly hair as these are adept at separating the curls to give definition without causing frizz.

When choosing combs and brushes, a certain amount of trial and error is to be expected before you find the right products for you. But once you find a comb or brush that suits your hair, you'll probably end up keeping it for life.

Tip 6: *Looking After Long Hair*

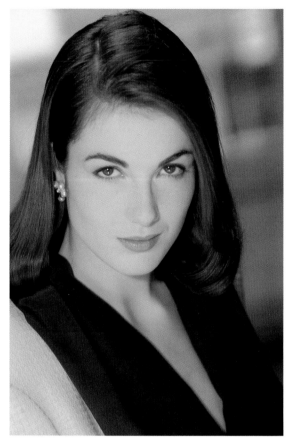

To keep long hair in peak condition takes time and dedication. However, if you are prepared to put some work into maintenance, long, glossy locks can look stunning. The number one enemy of long hair is heat. The tips of your hair are probably about four years old, and four years of regular treatment with hair-dryers and various electrical styling appliances may result in some damage.

Be aware that long hair is heavy on products, needing far more shampoo and conditioner than, say, a short bob. The ends need regular, possibly daily conditioning with a specialized conditioning oil to keep split ends at bay. One of the main problems with long hair is split ends, which can't be mended, but rather, have to be cut away. A regular trim every six weeks can be the solution.

It's important not to brush long hair when it is wet as this can tear the hair. Using a wide-toothed comb to brush out any post-washing tangles is

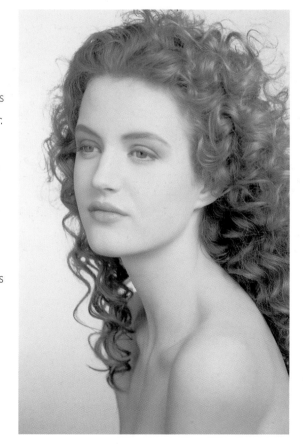

much gentler on the shafts and less likely to cause trauma to the hair. A wide paddle brush is the best brush for long hair, effectively allowing hair's natural oils to coat all the way down to the very ends. Stylists often recommend keeping long hair all one length for optimum shine and effect. Long hair also has a tendency to become static and flyaway; remedies for this include using a serum after conditioning, allowing a longer drying time to let the hair dry naturally, and investing in an "ionic" brush that generates negative ions to smooth the hair shaft.

Tip 7: *Curling & Straightening Hair*

With so many innovative styling tools to choose from, you can create a variety of looks with relative ease, especially as many tools now even come with a DVD or booklet explaining how to get different looks.

Any styling that involves heat or chemicals will, however, cause damage to hair over a period of time. Black women with tight, curly locks can have their hair "relaxed" – a chemical treatment that straightens out those tight curls. Although this gives greater flexibility for styling, it can leave hair weakened and prone to breakage. You should always visit a professional salon for this rather than attempting it yourself at home. Relaxed hair should always be well conditioned and brushed with a wide-toothed comb to avoid tangling. More recently invented nonchemical relaxing systems are thought to be less effective, and need to be repeated more often.

To cut down on the risks of styling damage, it is essential not to skimp on your styling tools. A curling iron with a plain, uncoated metal barrel might be cheap but will play havoc with your hair's condition. Always look for ceramic-coated curling irons, or straightening irons that quickly reach a high heat without scorching your hair; these will lock in, rather than leach out, the natural oils. Hairstylists recommend always using a heat protection spray to minimize heat damage, such as dryness, frizziness or split ends. The most recent innovation is the use of crushed tourmaline in straightening irons, allowing more ions to smooth and reduce static. Ionic technology is designed to generate a field of negative particles that break apart water molecules into smaller ones, more easily absorbed into hair for more moisture and less brittleness. Ionic brushes and styling tools can improve your hair's condition. So called wet-to-dry straightening tools can be used on wet hair to dry and straighten at the same time. However, no matter how many precautions are taken, these tools dry out hair very quickly, leading to damage. They are best saved for occasional use.

There are many products available to support your styling methods: specialized hair oils to use with straightening and curling irons; smoothing balms to give a sleeker result, and leave-in conditioners and serums that can help to keep hair frizz-free for longer. A successful styling session is a combination of good tools and the right products to help maintain your look. When first using a straightening or curling iron you'll need to practice to get the look you want, but be patient and don't expect a salon result the first time!

If you want to have a perm, remember that this is not something to attempt on damaged hair. Don't perm and tint within the same two weeks, and don't perm if you have an irritated scalp. Always use a conditioner each time you wash permed hair, and avoid brushing if possible, as this will pull out the curl.

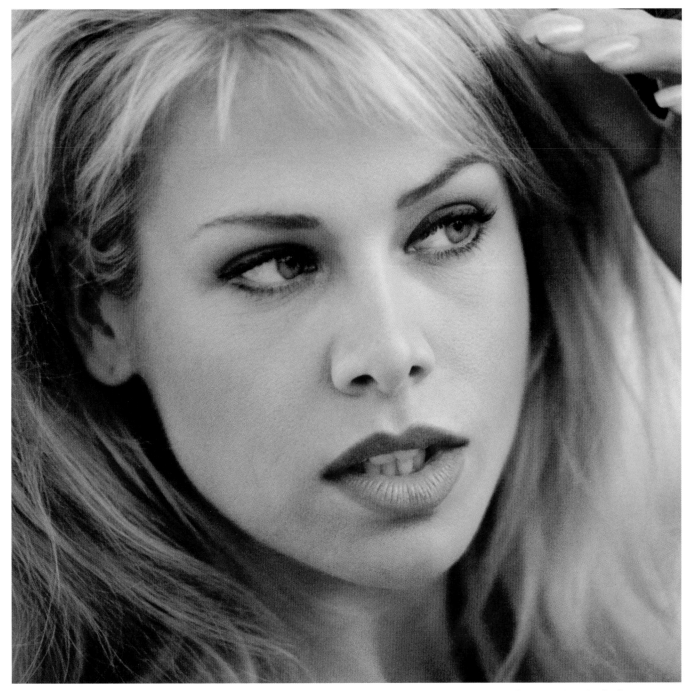

Styling tools that involve the application of chemicals or heat can damage your hair, especially when used regularly. To reduce the risk of inflicting long-term damage on your hair, invest in high-quality styling products.

Tip 8: *Dry Hair*

Dry hair is hair that doesn't contain enough moisture. It lacks shine, tangles easily and feels rough. There are many causes of dry hair, such as environmental damage from the sun, and chemical damage from the use of harsh colorants or perming. In normal hair, very little water can get in or out of the shaft because the hair cuticles are undamaged. In dry hair, however, the cuticle has become damaged and allows the hair to be porous, offering little or no protection from outside factors. The damage, unless halted, worsens over time. For tightly curled hair, salon steam treatments are excellent, infusing the hair with moisture.

If your hair has a constant tendency to break, apparently for none of the reasons detailed above, check with your doctor; the cause may be prescription drugs or a nutritional imbalance.

Washing & Conditioning

Washing dry hair will not strip it of its natural oils. Whatever your hair type, your prime objective must be to keep the hair clean; and if you use the correct products, gently massaged into the scalp, you will be able to restore shine to even the driest hair. Always choose a shampoo and conditioner that is suitable for dry hair. Look out for products that use the words "conditioning," "humectant" (meaning drawing moisture to the hair) or "moisturizing," as these tend to have more hydrating properties in them and leave a fine coating on the hair to make it more manageable. Try to deeply condition your hair at least once a week. There are specialized products available, often using warm oil, to give dry hair an intense treatment. It's also a good idea to look for alcohol-free shampoo and conditioners as alcohol content can cause drying.

Styling & Drying

Those with dry hair should keep any form of styling – straightening, curling and blow-drying, for example – to an absolute minimum, as any processing has the potential to dry hair out even further. Having any dry and split ends professionally trimmed out regularly will help keep hair looking less dry. Use a serum to smooth down the cuticle shafts to keep hair looking defined and glossy. Keep hair covered with a hat or scarf when in strong sunshine to avoid further dehydration.

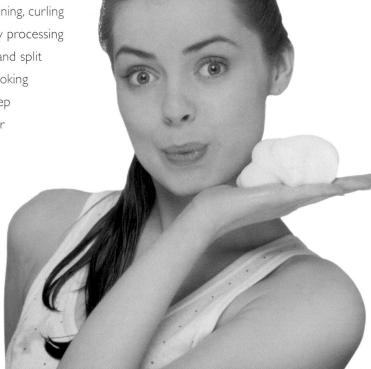

Styling hair with products such as mousse and sprays can lead to dry, damaged hair. If you do use these products, it is especially important that you rehydrate your hair with some of the methods described here.

Tip 9: *Split Ends & Breaks*

At some time in their lives, most women will suffer from hair breakage or split ends. While hormonal factors do come into play – during pregnancy or menopause, for example, on the whole it is environmental damage, overstyling and using harsh products that are to blame. Breaks and splits can never be mended; your hair will need a good professional cut and regular trimming until new growth has replaced damaged hair. In the meantime, however, there are steps you can take to disguise the worst of the damage and measures you can apply to stop future damage.

Avoiding Damage

Following a basic hair routine that involves staying away from styling or straightening tools, using cleansing and conditioning products that are alcohol-free and getting regular professional cuts are all critical for keeping hair soft, shiny and healthy. But it is not always practical to be such a hair purist! As with anything, moderation is key, and a certain amount of styling shouldn't prove too much of a problem.

Dealing with Existing Split Ends & Hair Breakage

The only way to be rid of split ends is to have them cut off. Hair breakage, though, could be the result of something as basic as being too rough with your hair while washing and towel-drying, or that your hairbrush is old and the bristle ends are no longer round and smooth. Gentleness is vital to hair health. Ionic technology in styling tools and dryers may help to improve hair condition, but another option is infrared technology. Some styling tools incorporate infrared for its ability to seal in moisture in the hair shaft, preventing dryness. Hair also feels softer and shinier as minimum moisture is taken out during the drying process.

If your hair is prone to breakage, this could be due to a number of factors. While it is possible that breakage is linked to a medical condition, it is more likely to be the result of

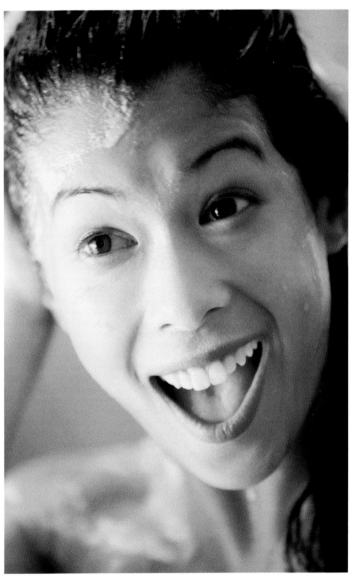

When washing youir hair, make sure you use cleansing and conditioning products that are alcohol-free.

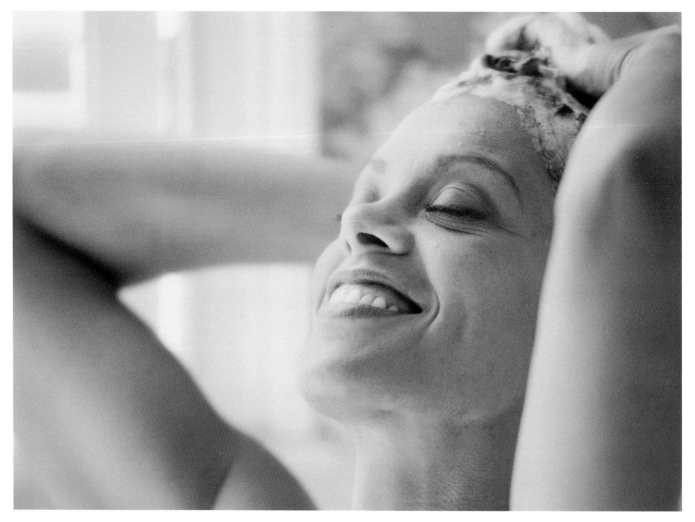

Special products are available for treating and preventing split ends. These intensive conditioners strengthen the hair by replenishing key amino acids.

perms, relaxing, extensions and bleaching. Anything that disturbs the hair's natural condition and growth can cause hair to be brittle, including blow-drying on a very hot setting. Black (African American) hair is particularly vulnerable to breakage due to its natural characteristics of being dry and tightly curled. Each twist of the hair can be a breaking point. It is recommended by experts that relaxing is not done more than once every 12 weeks. There are more and more specialized products available for hair that suffers from breakage, and these are mainly intense conditioners that replenish key amino acids to make the strands stronger.

Gentle towel-drying is essential for fragile hair – no scrubbing and tugging, and avoiding any hot hair appliances will be of great benefit. Intense conditioning treatments are essential. If your hair is extremely brittle, breaking often, and not responding to conditioning treatments, you should consult your doctor.

Tip 10: *Oily Hair*

The problem of oily hair is purely caused by a buildup of natural secretions known as sebum. Emitted from sebaceous glands in the scalp, sebum passes into the hair follicle and lies on the hair shafts. At certain times, such as puberty, sebum production increases. You should watch your diet and keep hydrated. Plenty of fresh fruit and salads with lots of water to drink will help.

Washing & Conditioning

A widely held fallacy is that frequent shampooing makes the hair even more greasy. In fact, oily hair responds well to regular washing, but it is important to use products specifically for your hair type. Shampoo for oily hair will clear away the grease without stripping the hair and making it feel dry. As the scalp produces the same amount of sebum regardless of hair style, short hair can often need more washing than medium or long hair. Using a gentle shampoo, you can wash as often as you like without encouraging more oil or damaging the hair. It is a good idea to condition the ends of the hair only as this won't overload the scalp. Look for shampoos that are "balancing" or "normalizing" as these will help to reduce sebum production.

Another very useful preparation for oily hair, especially when it is fine and flyaway, is a light hair gel or mousse. Even if you let your hair dry naturally after applying it, you will find that it gives extra bounce and shine.

Drying & Styling

Oily hair can often look dull and lifeless, so styling and blow-drying are ideal ways of giving it back some movement and body. Like any hair type, however, try to give your tresses a break from styling now and then. While the newer hair nearer the scalp will look better from blow-drying, the older hair nearer the bottom can be just as prone to split ends as dry hair. Try to hold back on styling products on oily hair as they just add to the overload.

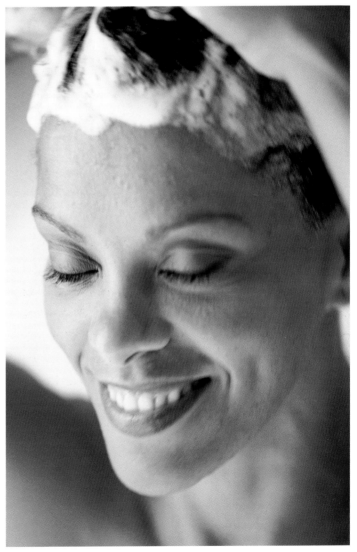

Oily hair responds well to regular washing, but you must choose the right products for your hair type.

Tip 11: *Dandruff*

Dandruff brings misery to those who suffer from this common, harmless, but distressing condition. The skin is constantly renewing itself – old cells fall away from the scalp as newer ones grow beneath. In those people with dandruff, this process happens very quickly so a large number of cells are shedding at any one time. Often, these flakes shed in large clumps visible to the human eye. It is very difficult to completely eradicate dandruff, but it can be kept under control. More severe dandruff is often caused by seborrheic dermatitis, causing greasy scales. You may find that dandruff is less severe during the summer months as sunlight inhibits the fungus responsible for dandruff.

Dandruff can be kept at bay by using shampoos that contain selenium sulfide or zinc oxide that contain active ingredients to fight dandruff. Severe dandruff will benefit from shampoos containing ketoconasole, as this is an antifungal that acts against the yeast-like fungus that causes seborrheic dermatitis. Shampoos and conditioners containing tea tree oil are also found to be effective as tea tree oil is a natural antifungal agent.

It is a myth that hair with dandruff doesn't need conditioning – once again, look for a specific antidandruff product that contains active ingredients to help fight against it. Some good bacteria on the scalp naturally fights against dandruff. Chemical hair dyes can destroy the good bacteria, so try to avoid coloring until your dandruff is well under control.

Make sure that your diet is a healthy one and includes white meat or fish, eggs, fresh fruits and raw vegetables. If dandruff persists, visit your doctor.

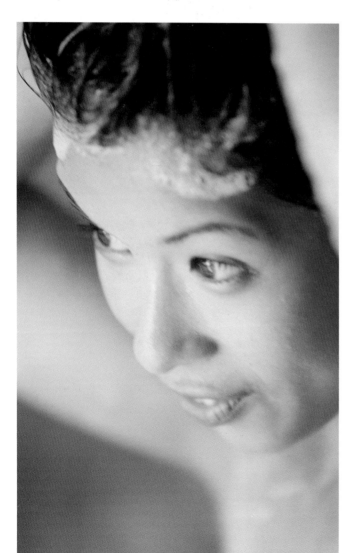

Special shampoos are available that will help treat a severe dandruff problem. If you only have a minor dandruff problem, try using shampoos and conditioners that contain tea tree oil, as it is a natural antifungal agent.

Tip 12: *Permed & Dyed Hair*

At some stage in their lives, most women experiment with different hair shades and styles, and luckily there are many ways to color and restyle your look. Hair dyes have received publicity in the past for their suggested links with cancer. Most concerns surround dark-colored, permanent dyes used every four to six weeks. The two chemicals scientists are particularly worried about are para-phenylenediamine and tetrahydro-6-nitroquinoxaline. These chemicals have been shown to damage the body's genetic material, and to cause cancer in animals. If you are concerned about using hair dye, it advisable to contact your doctor, particularly if you are pregnant or are trying to become preganant.

Permanent Hair Color

This is a process best done by professionals. Permanent home-dye disasters are notoriously difficult to correct! If you choose a permanent dye, you are committed to re-visiting your hairdressing salon every six to eight weeks; more if you find that your roots show more quickly. Choosing a soft or subtle shade will decrease the chance of roots growing very obviously. A permanent dye is not a cheap solution, but it can be dramatic and enhancing.

Highlights and Lowlights

Highlights and lowlights are designed to boost your natural color and give it more interest and reflectiveness. Highlights, lighter than your natural color, brighten and illuminate the hair and can give hair a fresh and sun-kissed appearance. Lowlights, darker than your natural color, add more depth and drama. Your colorist will dye only small strands of hair equally over your head, rather than do an overall flat, one-color dye.

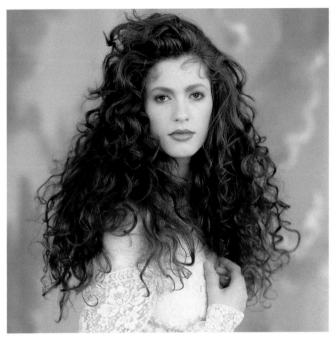

There are a number of ways to dye your hair. Choose the right one for you, depending on the look you are after and how long you want it to last.

Semipermanent Dye

Semipermanent dyes are a block color, with no natural highlights or variations and can be a good way of experimenting with different shades. Lasting between 10 and 20 washes before the color is fully erased, the color fades with each wash.

Temporary Dye

Available at drug stores, temporary colors are a fun way to change your hair color until your next wash. Temporary dyes are unable to lighten your hair; they only darken. Always try a skin patch test 24 hours before applying to check for allergic reactions.

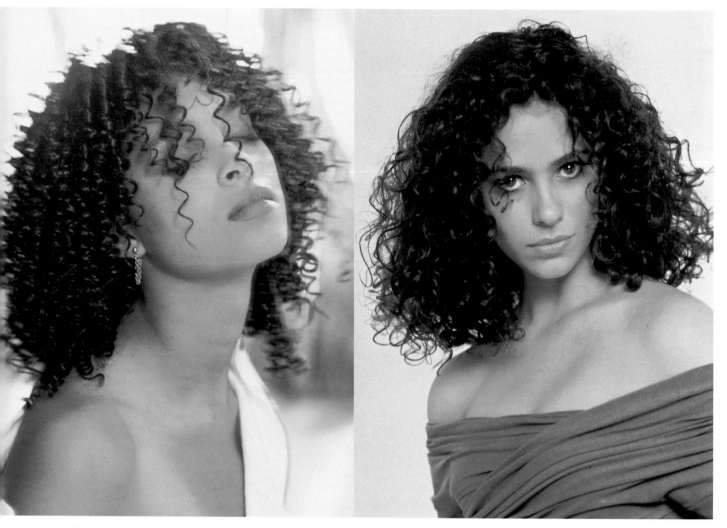

A good perm by an expert can really help to add body to lifeless and unmanageable hair.

Perming

Lovely, bouncing, loose-curl perms can give your hair a contemporary and incredibly natural appearance, and advanced techniques mean that perms are gentler than ever before.

Make an effort to improve the condition of your hair before a perm if it is at all out of shape, as hair that is brittle and dry will not respond well to perming. Ensure that you deeply condition several times prior to a treatment. Perms work best on medium and long hair, which has more flexibility in terms of styling. Perms can give body to fine, flyaway hair and also retexturize coarse, unmanageable hair. Even curly hair can stand a perm to tame curls into a more even style.

Don't even contemplate a home perm – although there are kits available. To get a good outcome, with the style and size of curl that you would like, it is imperative to consult an expert. As there are many products available for permed hair, ensure you choose one that offers good conditioning to support your new curls.

The perm is a two-stage process. The first lotion applied is a chemical that softens the structure of the hair; this is then rinsed away very thoroughly and the second lotion is applied. This is a neutralizer that sets the hair into the new position determined by the curling rods. A final rinse and the perm is complete.

Tip 13: *Pregnancy and Hair*

While many women enjoy thicker, shinier hair during pregnancy, due to hormonal surges and possibly a more careful diet, as many women will experience hair loss, dryness and breakage. There has been much media coverage about the safety of hair dyes during pregnancy, and although there is little hard and fast evidence that it can affect an unborn baby, many women choose not to dye their hair at this time. If you have any concerns about this, it is advisable to consult with your doctor. If you continue to dye your hair, be aware that during pregnancy hair can be more porous, and therefore the results more unpredictable.

If you find that your hair is more brittle during pregnancy, invest in nutritious conditioners and check that your diet includes enough protein. As hair breakage tends to occur nearer the top of the head than the bottom, smoothing styling products can cover the evidence, helping the shafts to lie flat, and making shorter strands look less obvious.

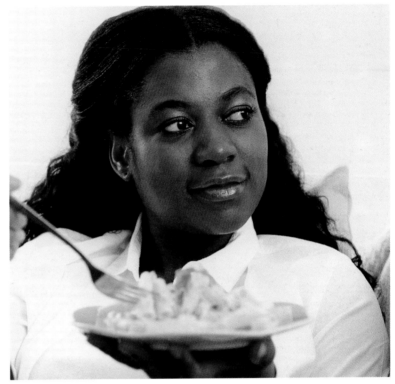

For healthy hair during pregnancy, ensure that you eat a balanced and nutritious diet that includes enough protein.

Hair loss tends to occur more commonly after the baby is born, and is a result of the loss of hormones that stopped your hair shedding at its normal rate. You should consult your doctor, however, if you find that your hair is becoming excessively thin.

During pregnancy, many women find that thanks to weight gain, the shape of their face can change, and a new style may suit your shape better than the old one. It is also a great professional tip to get a low-maintenance haircut when you are pregnant, as once the baby is born, trips to the hairdresser may become harder to fit in!

Some pregnant women find that their perm loses its bounce. Nothing can be done about this, but a healthy diet will ensure that the hair regains its former condition soon after the birth.

Tip 14: *Teenage Hair*

Teenagers are bombarded with hormonal changes and disturbances during puberty, and these changes can have a direct effect on hair. Normally, this shows itself as an overproduction of sebum, or oil, in the hair, leading to lank and greasy locks; the same hormones responsible for acne cause this.

As puberty progresses, this overproduction will settle down, but can lead to self-consciousness and stress. The only way to deal with teen hair is to wash it — regularly! By washing away the excess oil, at least once or even twice a day, hair will become more manageable and clean. Look for hair products that specifically tackle oily hair.

Hair experts often advise teens against perming as their hair is in a transient stage and the results are variable. While teens love to experiment with styling gels and waxes, it is advisable to always wash the hair thoroughly after use to avoid creating product buildup to add to the grease. To remove waxes and gels, look for shampoos that are "detoxifying" as these are more effective on the oil bases used in styling products. Better still, search out products that are labeled "oil free."

Diet is also an important consideration for teengaers, as this will have an impact on the amount of oil produced. Eat a balanced diet that is low in fats and sugars. Consume plenty of fresh fruit and vegetables and avoid fast food and convenience foods. Also, make sure you drink plenty of water, as this will help keep hair hydrated and looking silky and shiny. All vitamins are important, but vitamin A is good for the skin and will encourage a healthy scalp.

It is essential for teenagers to wash their hair regularly to guard against greasy, oily locks. Perms like this are usually best avoided, as the results can be variable.

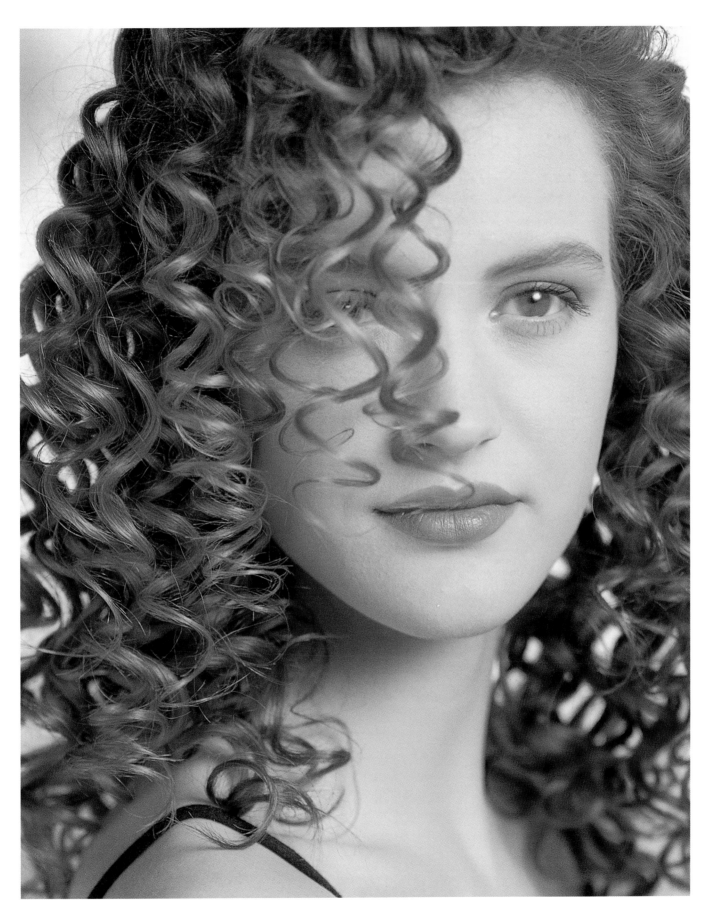

Tip 15: *Unwanted Facial Hair*

Facial hair can be a very distressing and embarrassing problem, and it generally worsens from the age of about 40, when women's bodies produce progressively less of the female hormone estrogen and more of the male hormone testosterone. The amount of facial hair you have is the result of several factors. First, the darker your skin tone, the more likely you are to grow dark, more obvious hairs. Second, if you have thick hair on your head, your body hair is likely to be similar. Third, side effects from medications such as steroids, antidepressants, or the birth control pill are all thought to be contributing factors.

Removal Methods

Waxing

Facial waxing strips are readily available at drug stores, but are felt by skin experts to be too harsh for the delicate upper lip area. Excessive pulling and stripping at the skin can cause trauma.

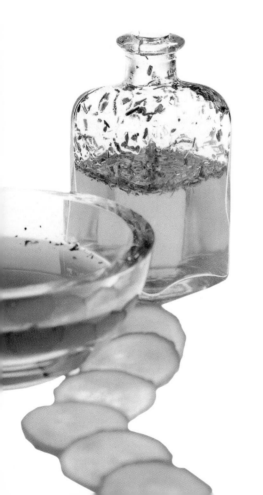

Depilatory Creams

These dissolve the hair from just below the surface of the skin using chemicals. Always patch test for allergies, and check that the product you use is suitable for the face.

Shaving

No expert would recommend shaving the delicate skin on a woman's face, no matter how serious. Soft and delicate skin is unable to cope with the abrasions of a razor.

Laser Hair Removal

This method uses a laser to deliver a high-intensity light providing heat energy. This heat damages or destroys the hair root, but is not effective on

Cucumber, lavender oil and tea tree oil are ideal ingredients for a homemade shaving lotion – they are three of nature's most effective skin soothers and will help to make the act of shaving a much more pleasant experience.

those with gray, white, blonde or light red hair as the laser targets pigment. A course of treatments is required.

Electrolysis

This method of hair removal passes a small amount of energy via a fine needle through the hair follicle. This produces heat which in turn destroys the root. A course of treatments is required.

Threading

This is a skilled and effective way of removing hair from the root. Threaders use lengths of looped cotton to catch and pull out the hairs.

Plucking

Plucking is a reliable method of removing hair – usually from the eyebrows. Don't overpluck the brows; stick to the natural lines, removing only strays.

Tip 16: *Unwanted Body Hair*

All the same methods as mentioned in Tip 15 are suitable for body hair removal, but the larger the area to treat, the more pricey it can become.

Waxing

Wax is available in either liquid form, which is heated, applied to the skin and then stripped away using a muslin or cloth strip, or in the form of waxing strips – pre-impregnated strips of strengthened paper. In the case of warm wax, if you attempt to do it yourself, be very careful not to overheat the wax. Always apply wax in the direction of the hair growth to limit the likelihood of ingrown hairs. Brazilian waxing – which removes all hair from the pubic region – should only be done professionally, due to the delicate nature of the skin.

Shaving

Shaving is a quick but temporary way to remove underarm and leg hair. Use a shaving lubricant to avoid taking the top layer of skin away.

Epilators

Electrical epilators use tweezing heads that rotate over the skin, removing hair as they go. Hair is pulled from the root, so it can be painful, particularly under the arms where there are sensitive glands.

Sugaring

Sugaring works on a similar principle to waxing and originated in the Middle East. A sticky sugar paste grips the hair, then it is rolled away, uprooting the hairs. It is thought to be less painful than waxing and is said to keep hairs at bay for longer, usually up to eight weeks. You can buy premade sugaring preparations from beauty supply stores and some drug stores, but it is also possible to make your own.

When shaving hair it is essential to use a good gel or foam so that you will not take the top layer of skin off and cause damage and irritation.

Tip 17: *Wigs, Extensions & Hairpieces*

Hair extensions were developed by Simon Forbes at the Antenna Salon in London, England, in the 1980s. They give instant length and can transform a short cut into long luxuriant locks in a matter of hours, Hair extensions use either human hair or synthetic fibers that bond to your own hair, and can create a new look for glamour or medical reasons. If using synthetic fiber extensions, they should be of a high grade, and should look and act like human hair – being light, airy and silky to the touch. Caring for hair extensions is a little different from caring for your normal hair, and following the aftercare tips from your salon very carefully is essential to make them last. Extensions can be curled or highlighted, but this should only be done professionally. Don't brush your extensions too harshly, and use a soft bristled brush. It is advisable to dry your hair thoroughly before sleeping, and to tie it up at night to avoid accidental pulling.

Wigs and hairpieces have a long history; indeed, they were worn by men and women in ancient Egypt. They reached their most extravagant during the late 17th century with musical boxes, ornaments and even singing birds intertwined with the hair. After a period of decline, hairpieces made a dramatic comeback in the 1960s. The advent of artificial fibers made it possible to mass-produce wigs and hairpieces so that every woman could change her hairstyle in minutes. Today, there are many different reasons that women choose to wear a wig or a hairpiece. It may be due to a medical condition that causes hair loss, they may have naturally very thin and wispy hair or it may be that they just like to create a change without a visit to the salon. Wigs and hairpieces are available in human or synthetic fiber and quality varies enormously, but a key consideration when choosing is to find one that flatters the shape of your face. Oval shaped faces are the most versatile, suiting almost all styles, but those with round faces should avoid bobs, which only serve to make the face even rounder. Long, thin faces tend not to suit long wigs as these will accentuate the facial length. When choosing a color to suit your skin tone, look for shades close to your own natural hair color. However, the joy of a wig or hairpiece is that you can have fun with them and go as wild and vibrant as you like! As a general rule of thumb, however, those with dark skin tones should steer clear of light hair, and those with light skin tones should steer clear of very dark hair. Both can make the face looked leached of color. Human hair and synthetic wigs and hairpieces should be washed with mild shampoos and conditioner, and hung to dry. A detangling spray, applied once the hair is dry, will help to keep tangles at bay. Both can also be styled just as your own hair can, and it is helpful in the case of a full wig to invest in a wig stand, which makes styling easier.

A huge variety of wigs and hairpieces are available today, in numerous styles and colors. When choosing a wig, the key consideration is whether it suits the shape of your face.

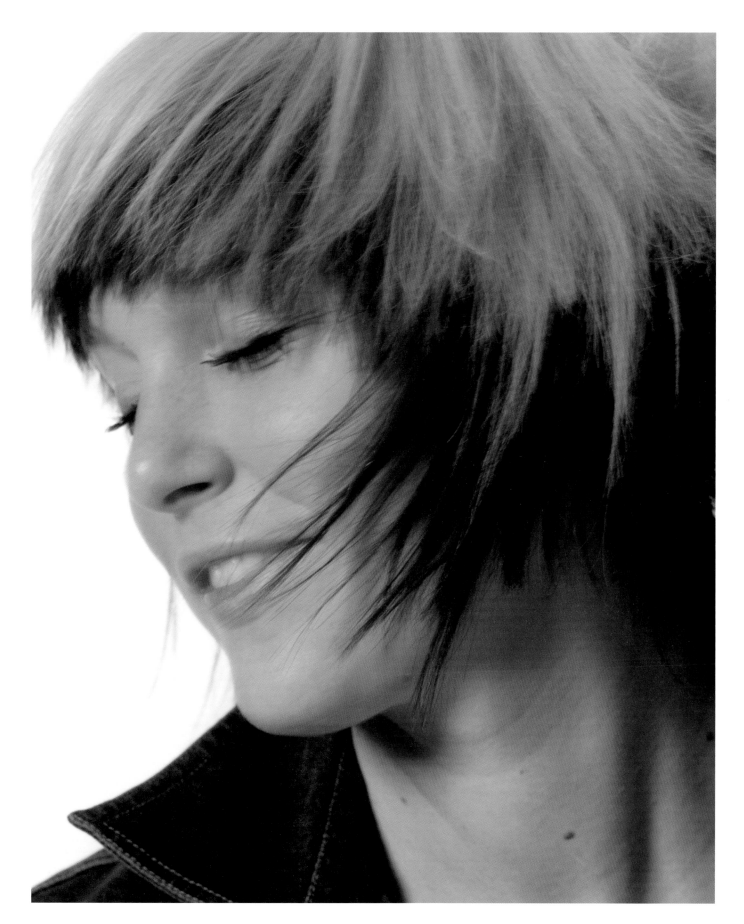

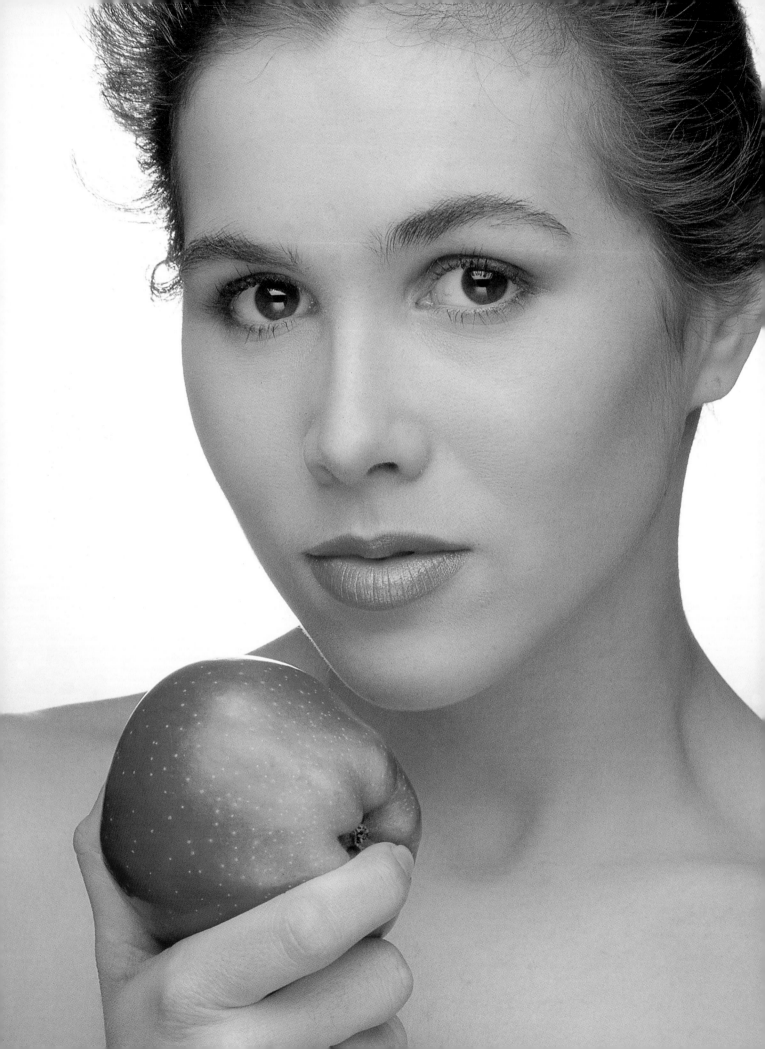

chapter two
HEALTHY SKIN

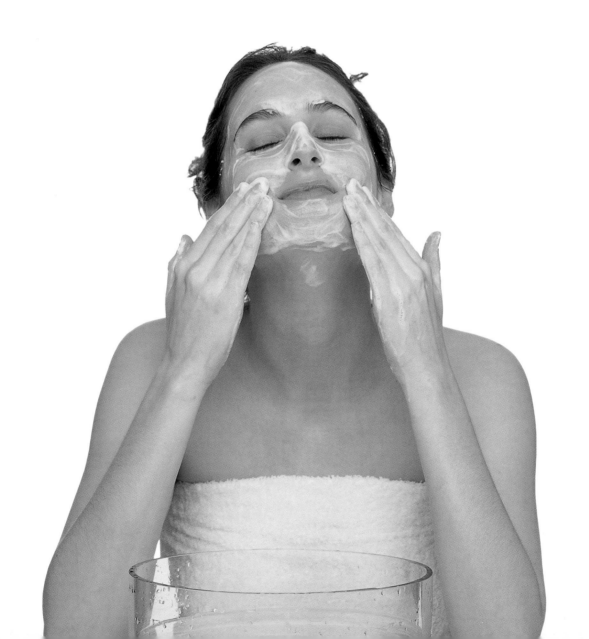

Tip 18: *Food for Beautiful Skin*

Skin is a living organ that covers the whole body. It is the body's largest organ, measuring about 16 square feet (1.5 m²). Its thickness varies from 1/500 inch (0.05 mm) on the eyelids, where it is at its most delicate and translucent, to 1/40 inch (0.65 mm) on the soles of the feet, where it is at its toughest. With the exception of the palms of the hands and the soles of the feet, the skin is covered with hair follicles.

It will be no surprise that what you put inside in terms of food very often has a direct reflection on the outside. Glowing, healthy skin is fed by a healthy diet.

Nutritionists recommend plenty of vitamin A for all around skin cell health. The best foods to provide your skin with this are dairy products – low-fat if you are watching your weight. Another key player in skin health is the group of foods that contain antioxidants, which fight against free radicals. Free radicals come from environmental pollutants such as sun exposure and smoking. Eating antioxidant rich foods will protect skin cells from disintegration and damage, and can have a direct effect on the look of your skin in both the long and short term. Foods rich in antioxidants include plums, artichokes, blueberries and pomegranates. Drinking green tea can also be a good source of antioxidants, and will also keep you well hydrated.

Essential fatty acids help to keep cell membranes healthy. As the cell membrane is responsible for holding water, this needs to be kept strong and healthy for skin to be hydrated, firm and more youthful in appearance. The best sources of these fatty acids are found in fish, nuts and oils.

A nutritious diet rich in vitamins and minerals is essential for healthy and attractive-looking skin. Eat plenty of fresh fruits and vegetables and avoid fatty fast foods and convenience foods.

Tip 19: *Know Your Skin Type*

Identifying your skin type is crucial to choosing the products that will give you the maximum benefits and results.

Normal Skin

This is neither too oily nor too dry and rarely gets blemish flare-ups. Pores are usually small and fine, and the texture of the skin is firm and supple.

Oily Skin

This type of skin tends to be shiny, particularly around the nose and chin areas where excess oil is often secreted. Blackheads and large pores are part of the oily skin condition. This type of skin is more common during hormonal changes such as puberty.

Dry Skin

This is the type of skin that is most prone to aging due to the lack of natural oils. Skin feels rough or tight, and there may be patches of obvious dry skin. Dry skin is generally not prone to breakouts.

Combination Skin

This type of skin is characterized by oiliness down the nose and across the forehead and chin. Occasionally, oiliness occurs at the hairline. Other skin areas are normal or slightly dry.

Sensitive Skin

Sensitive skin reacts to weather conditions, can feature redness and broken capillaries and often suffers irritated reactions to beauty products and makeup.

Problem Skin

It is invariably caused by acne – flare-ups of pimples, pus-filled sore spots and blackheads that don't easily heal. These can cause facial scarring. It is often over-oily.

A wealth of natural beauty products for different skin types are available, using everything from natural oils, honey and yogurt to fruits and vegetables. Always ensure you pick the right treatment for your skin type.

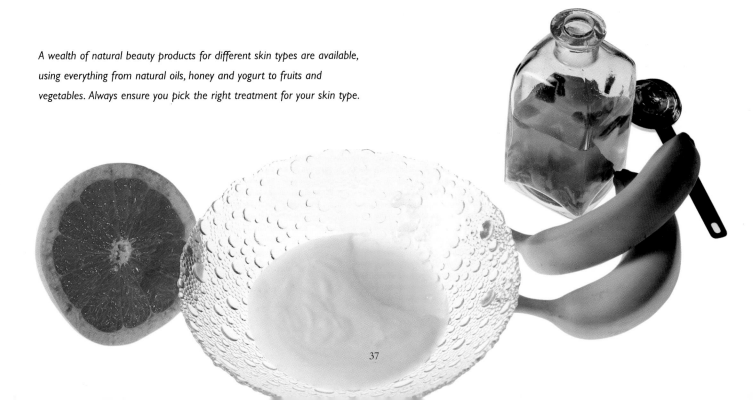

Tip 20: *Skin Cleansing*

Cleaning your skin is one of the key ways to maintain a healthy complexion. It removes traces of grime and makeup, and is a gentle way to rid the skin of old cells to reveal fresher, newer ones beneath. Without cleansing, skin can look dull and gray, particularly if you live in a city where air pollution is high. Even when your complexion feels clean, after a day there will be a buildup of sweat and dirt that can lead to clogged pores, blemishes and blackheads. So a good night and morning cleansing routine can give you a rosy, smooth complexion.

Cleansing should be the first step of your skin care routine. It should be thorough, but it should also be gentle. A light, easy-to-smooth formula is ideal. Warm it in the palm of your hand first, then massage it gently into the skin before wiping it off with a soft facial tissue or cotton ball. Never drag the skin.

Oily Skin

Oily skin types should stick to oil-free lotions or mild foaming cleansers, as these won't add more oil to the skin.

Dry Skin

Dry skin types benefit most from cleansing creams, which consist of a high level of oil and lower water combinations to leave skin feeling supple.

Sensitive Skin

Sensitive skin types react best to cleansing milks with a balanced oil and water content that are gentle and nonabrasive.

Don't clean your face with soap as it is highly alkaline (skin is naturally acidic) and will strip away facial oils, breaking down natural protection.

Oils such as jojoba and grapeseed are rich in vitamins and minerals. They will both cleanse and moisturize the skin effectively without making it too greasy.

Tip 21: *Deep Cleansing*

Make time to give your skin a very thorough, deep cleanse to get it really glowing and smooth. A cheap and effective way is to gently steam your face by pouring hot (not boiling) water in a bowl; add an essential oil to make it extra pampering, and position your face under a towel over the water. Allow 10 minutes or so for the hot steam to open up the pores, then massage your regular cleanser gently into your skin, paying particular attention to your forehead, nose and chin. Remove with a clean, warm, damp cloth or cotton pads, ensuring that you do not drag the skin. A weekly steam treatment will help to keep your skin free from blackheads and blemishes. It is particularly important for oily skin, but do not perform more than once every two weeks if you have dry skin, which tends to be more delicate.

Clay masks are extremely effective in drawing out any impurities, particularly around problem areas. As the clay dries, it shrinks, pulling away blackheads and dead skin cells from the opened pores. It is extremely important, however, to close the pores after this process to stop more debris accumulating. Use either a good splash of cold water or a toner formulated to your skin type, but be aware that using water can make your skin feel temporarily tight. Skin really does look glowing and fresh after this treatment, but don't be tempted to overdo it; once a week is sufficient.

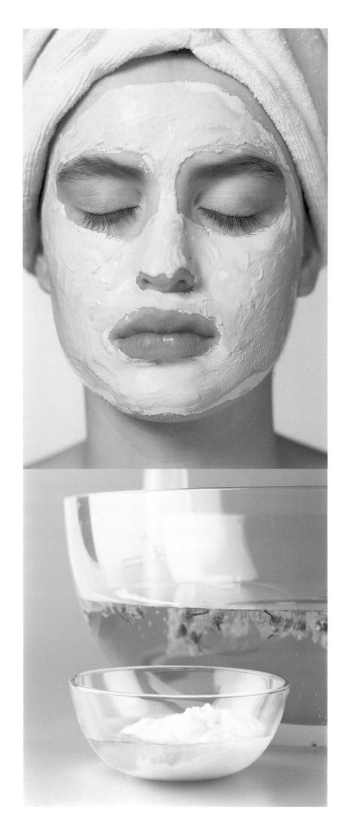

Top: Face masks are a very effective way of removing impurities. Bottom: Steam cleansing your face with a herbal infusion will increase the efficacy of the steam and leave your skin clean, refreshed and glowing.

Tip 22: *Choosing a Moisturizer*

A moisturizer is defined as a mix of chemical or natural agents designed to make skin softer and more flexible by increasing its hydration. The sky is the limit when it comes to how much money you can spend on this one beauty item alone! But price doesn't necessarily reflect results, and picking the perfect moisturizer for you will pay off over and over in terms of the comfort and look of your skin. Regular moisturizing should begin in your teens.

Moisturizer keeps water locked in the skin's cells by helping to reinforce the thin, oily layer on the surface of the skin, known as the hydrolipidic film – literally, water-oil film. This film is vital in preventing moisture from being lost through the skin, and in keeping the skin smooth, supple and youthful. Applying moisturizer is also a good opportunity to massage the skin, which helps to stimulate blood circulation and increase muscle tone.

The manufacturers of moisturizers are in a competitive market, and the variation can be baffling as they struggle to find a point of difference to give you "younger looking" skin. However, the bottom line is that while complex ingredients can make a subtle difference, all your skin really wants is to feel soft, comfortable and well hydrated, and water contained in moisturizers will plump up the cells making lines less obvious. It's a good idea to get as many samples as possible to see how the different brands suit your skin. What is one woman's elixir of youth is another woman's allergy!

All skin has its own natural moisturizing ability, but as we grow older this decreases. All skin types should moisturize morning and night to keep a constant feed of hydration. Older skin will benefit

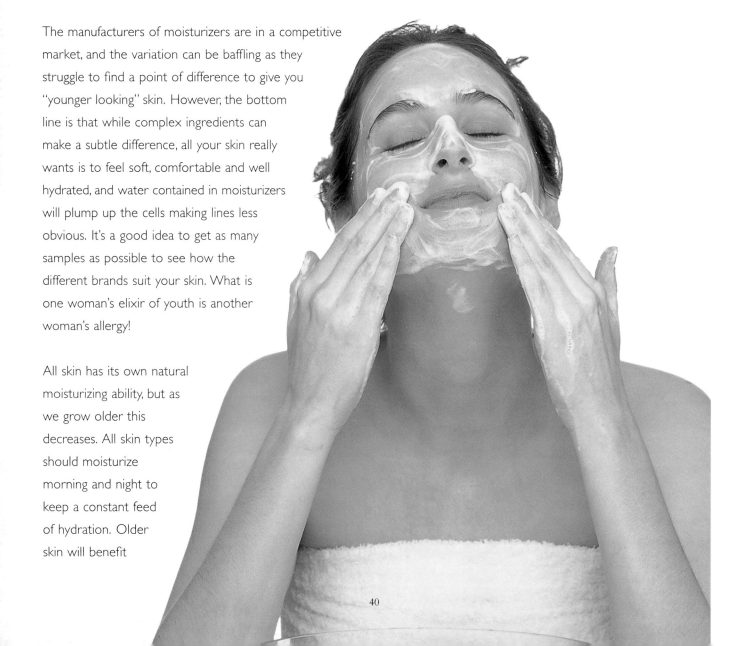

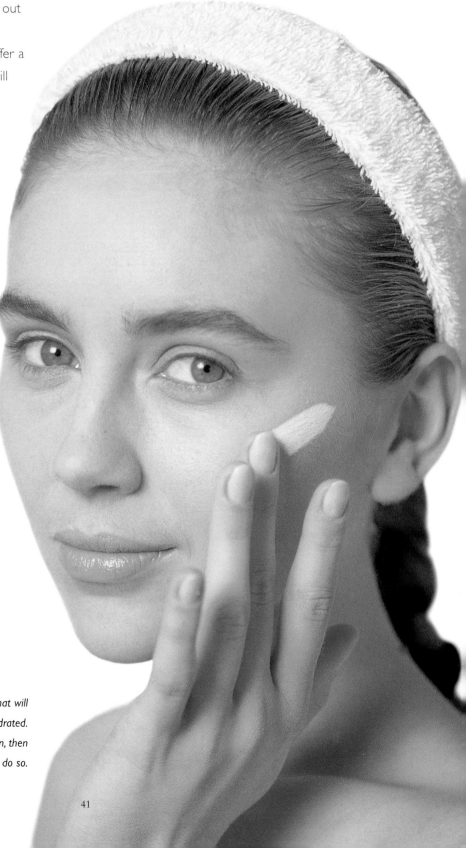

from an increased level of moisture to plump out wrinkles, and there are now more products specifically targeted at "mature" skin. These offer a more heavy duty moisturization, but should still be easily absorbed and not feel sticky on the surface of the skin. Young skin may well need hydration, but doesn't benefit from any added agents that offer to plump or firm out wrinkles. As skin behaves differently at different life stages, you may find you need to switch; for example, if your skin is going through an oily phase, the last thing it needs is more oil, but it will still benefit from moisturization. In this case, an oil-free moisturizer will pay off. Luckily, most available moisturizers are labeled with their skin type specific abilities, so as long as you correctly identify your skin type, the supporting moisturizer will act in conjunction with it. The one crucial ingredient, however, regardless of age or skin type, is sunscreen. The sun, direct or indirect, is responsible for rapid skin aging and wrinkling.

The skin around the eyes is thinner than on any other part of the body, so special care is required when choosing and applying moisturizer in this area.

Left: Moisturizing facial washes are available that will cleanse the skin and help to keep it hydrated.
Right: When applying moisturizer, dab it onto the skin, then gently massage it in. Try not to drag the skin when you do so.

Tip 23: *Avoiding Harmful Ingredients*

Beauty products are stringently tested and have to adhere to intensive health and safety codes before they can be used on human skin. Therefore, it is unlikely that your beauty routine can actually be harmful. However, by their very nature, unless you choose specifically organic and all-natural products, beauty products are heavily comprised of chemicals, artificial colorings and fragrances. It's worth remembering, though, that chemicals in makeup and skin care products don't just sit on your skin – they can be absorbed into your body, and there is little evident research into what the long-term impact of these chemicals might be. While the amount of potentially harmful ingredients may be small, over a lifetime they can add up. Fans of organic (meaning produced without chemical intervention, such as pesticides) beauty products will often say, "If you wouldn't put it on your plate, why put it on your skin?"

Key ingredients that are subject to scrutiny are parabens. Used as a preservative to prolong the shelf life of makeup and skin care products, these are considered to be a cause for concern by ethical groups for their potential hormone disrupting links. Parabens are relatively easy to identify on labeling, with common terms including "propylparaben" or "butylparaben." A notable labeling offence is the use of the word "natural." Often, the word "natural" is absolutely meaningless. This term, when used on cosmetic ingredient listings, could equally apply to petroleum derivatives as plants. Phthalates, (pronounced without the "ph") is a chemical family sometimes found in PVC plastics to soften them, and which has been linked by studies to reproductive damage. In cosmetic use, phthalates add flexibility and give an oily, moisturizing film. They can be used to make the alcohol in perfumes unpalatable and enhance fragrance and color. However, study findings vary, and there is little information on long-term use.

It has been estimated that 95 percent of chemicals used in cosmetics are derived from the petroleum industry. A good proportion of allergic reactions to makeup, which can range from minor skin irritation such as redness or itchiness, to severe flaking and peeling skin, are caused by "perfume" – a labeling umbrella term for up to as many as 80 unlisted ingredients, making it very difficult to pinpoint the exact culprit of a reaction. Bear in mind that there is no skin benefit to perfume in skin care products and cosmetics.

If you have allergies to skin care products and makeup, or you are ethically concerned about the composition of your brands, try to choose your makeup and skin care products from companies that are committed to avoiding potentially harmful ingredients. There is an increasingly large range to choose from.

Alternatively, it is possible to make your own treatments at home using a range of natural ingredients including essential oils and fruits and vegetables. If you decide to do this, please follow the advice from a professional or from a trusted textbook. It is not advisable to make your own treatments if you do not know what you are doing.

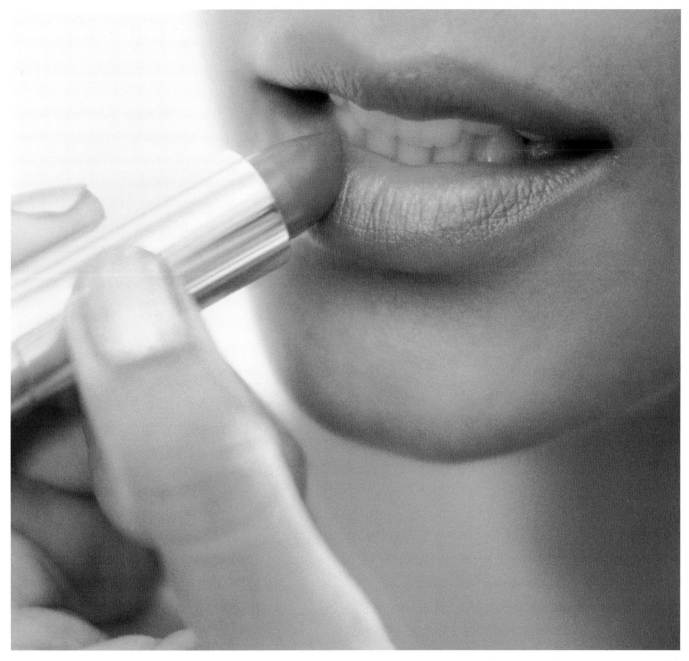

Beauty products and cosmetics are tested thoroughly before they are allowed to be sold, but some people do fear what the long-term consequences of regular use might be. There are an increasing number of products available that do not use potentially harmful ingredients.

Tip 24: *Exfoliating*

Exfoliating is a method of using tools or creams that are abrasive and will slough away dead skin cells, revealing newer, fresher ones beneath. It can greatly enhance the appearance of your skin, both on your face and body, by improving circulation and allowing better absorption of oils and creams. In fact, everyone exfoliates naturally as the body loses thousands of tiny skin cells every minute. Manual or chemical exfoliation simply speeds up the process. Natural skin regeneration decreases with age so while a teenager is unlikely to need to exfoliate, by the time we are in our 40s, the process has significantly slowed. This can lead to skin looking dull and grayish. Darker skin tones are particularly affected as the dead cells can look pale, making a marked contrast to fresher, dark skin.

Picking a method of exfoliating purely comes down to personal choice. Using manual scrubs such as sisal or nylon are quick, and effective while taking a bath or shower. They will always need a lubricating agent, such as mild soap, to avoid being too harsh on the skin and leaving scratch marks. Dry skin brushing is very effective, but has the drawback of leaving a flurry of cells on the floor! A sponge, used dry or wet, can be used to perform very gentle exfoliation as the material naturally loosens old cells.

There is a vast array of equipment for scrubbing, rubbing and exfoliating various parts of the body. Don't be overwhelmed by the selection; it is simply that certain tools are better on partidular parts of the body. When deciding what to buy, look first at those made from natural fibers, which tend to be gentler on the skin than artificial materials. It is important to keep exfoliating equipment clean and dry when not in use, because bacteria can grow among the damp fibers. Nylon scrubs have the advantage of being machine-washable.

An exfoliating product such as a salt scrub works in the same way as the tools, but feel more luxurious and pampering. They literally whisk away cell debris using abrasive grains. Often these grains, including walnut shell, coconut husk or salt and sugar, are soaked in oils that moisturize the skin at the same time, and leave the skin feeling silky and super soft. AHA (alpha hydroxy acid) based exfoliating products sound more scary than they actually are! These smooth the skin by dissolving cells away from the skin's surface, and if used correctly can be extremely safe. Always follow instructions carefully. When exfoliating your face, you should use a product designed specifically for the more fragile facial skin.

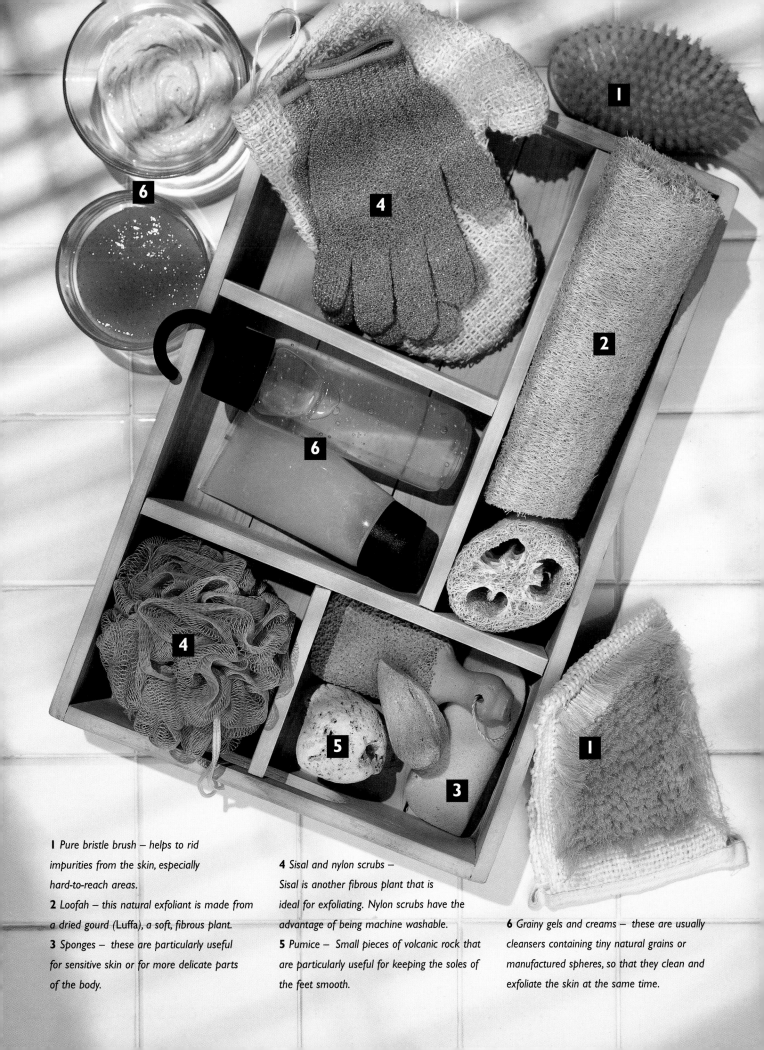

1 Pure bristle brush – helps to rid impurities from the skin, especially hard-to-reach areas.

2 Loofah – this natural exfoliant is made from a dried gourd (Luffa), a soft, fibrous plant.

3 Sponges – these are particularly useful for sensitive skin or for more delicate parts of the body.

4 Sisal and nylon scrubs – Sisal is another fibrous plant that is ideal for exfoliating. Nylon scrubs have the advantage of being machine washable.

5 Pumice – Small pieces of volcanic rock that are particularly useful for keeping the soles of the feet smooth.

6 Grainy gels and creams – these are usually cleansers containing tiny natural grains or manufactured spheres, so that they clean and exfoliate the skin at the same time.

Tip 25: *What You Don't Need*

What your skin wants is to feel comfortable, pliable, soft and smooth, both on the face and body. Wild claims are made by beauty product manufacturers, each promising to be more anti-aging, more plumping and more beneficial than the others. Those connected with so-called "studies" are usually tested in very controlled circumstances in small groups so cannot necessarily be relied upon. But deciding what you feel is necessary for your skin is purely a personal choice. One thing is for sure, however: you don't need to spend a fortune on your beauty regime. There is no guarantee that even if you do splurge on an expensive cream, that it will have any added benefit to your skin than a more reasonably priced one. Some luxury creams have turned out to be far too rich for many women's skin, and ended up an expensive disappointment. The jury is still out on whether eye creams are truly a necessity. Many experts feel that although the skin around the eye area is delicate, it doesn't actually need a specific cream, but reacts just as well to a general purpose facial moisturizer. Ultimately, it is better to have fewer items that suit your skin well, than a plethora of different lotions and potions that have little or no effect.

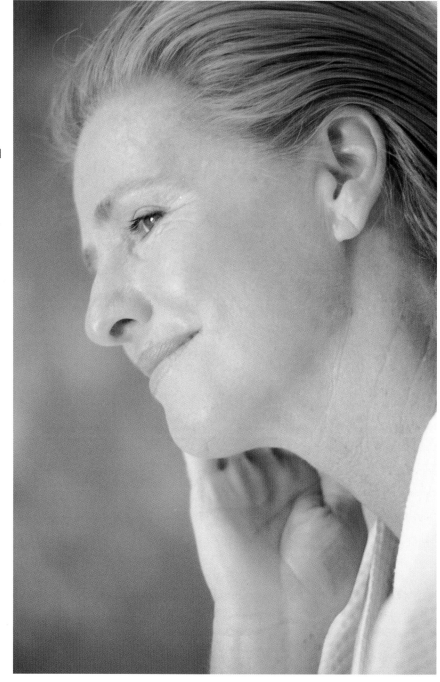

There is no need to spend a fortune on beauty products. Expensive creams are often no better than moderately priced ones.

46

Tip 26: *Daily Skin Protection*

If there is one beauty tip to pass on to your friends, it's this one. Always, always use skin care products that contain suncreen. Although black skin has a higher natural tolerance to the sun due to its genetic makeup, it still needs protecting. When the sun's ultraviolet rays reach the skin, in order to protect itself, the surface of the skin produces melanin – or a tan. While UVA rays are less intense than UVB, skin protection should block out both types. UVA rays are responsible for the premature aging of the skin, as well as the development of skin cancer, while UVB rays are the main cause of sunburn and skin cancer. Naturally, in the summer, when the sun is hotter, more damage is likely to be caused. Wearing a sunscreen with a sun protection factor (SPF) of at least 15 is essential to lessen the effects of the sun, both in terms of health and beauty. The rule of thumb is the more intense the sun, the higher the factor needed. A daily moisturizer containing sunscreen and antioxidants will protect it from environmental damage such as cigarette smoke, smog and pollutants, as well as keeping it soft and supple, but it does not offer sufficient protection against the harmful effects of the sun.

As well as using high-factor sunscreen on your skin, it is also a good idea to stay out of the strong sunlight between noon and 3 p.m. on hot days, and when you do venture out, ensure that vulnerable areas such as the back of your neck and your nose are protected. Use a waterproof sunblock or reapply after swimming. Watch out for the appearance of new moles or changes in existing ones – this can be a sign of skin cancer.

When relaxing by the pool or on the beach in the summer, it is essential that you protect your skin with high-factor sunscreen, and it is also a good idea to wear a hat to give your head and face additional protection.

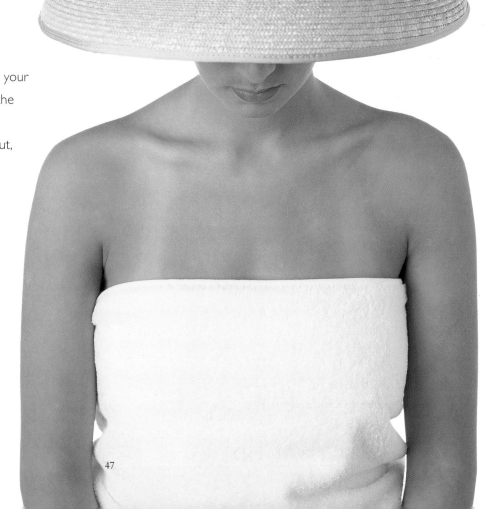

Tip 27: *Coping with Dry Skin*

Like normal skin, dry skin has an enviably fine texture, but it also tends to be thin and prone to varicose veins. There is insufficient sebum to keep the skin nourished, and without additional care, dry skin has a tendency to become rough and flaky, leading to fine lines and premature wrinkles. Dry skin types tend to suffer in any weather conditions, so it is essential to moisturize correctly all year round. Although everyone should drink plenty of water, those with dry skin need to take more care with this than most. When choosing a moisturizer for dry skin, look out for the word "humectant" on the packaging. Humectants draw moisture to the skin, so are an added bonus. There is a wide range of skin oils – usually containing plant extracts – both for face and body that dry skin types can benefit hugely from. Using a specialized oil under a dry skin moisturizer will give more comfort and suppleness, especially at night. Dry skin types benefit hugely from exfoliation so that your moisturizer directly freshens new cells once the old ones have been sloughed away. It's a mistake, though, to think that an abrasive exfoliator is better. Dry skin needs to be treated gently, especially on the face. Keep a jar of your favorite moisturizer in your desk drawer at work, or in your purse so you can give your skin on-the-spot relief, and where there is air-conditioning or central heating, be extra vigilant about applying.

Applying oils to problem areas offers an effective treatment for dry skin. There is a wide range of skin oils available for both the face and the body, most of which contain plant extracts that will hydrate problem areas.

Tip 28: *Coping with Oily Skin*

Oily skin produces more sebum than it needs, which means that the skin will have fewer wrinkles, but a tendency to blackheads and acne as the pores become blocked. The skin itself is often thick and the pores large. Despite all this, oily skin needs moisture in the same way as any other skin type, but what it doesn't need is more oil. Washing your face morning and night with a skin-type-specific facial wash can help cut down on sebum production. Moisturizers that don't contain oil are best for oily skin as they won't overload the glands that produce sebum. For coping strategies during the day, especially in warm weather, look out for oil blotters: small sheets of paper that will fit in your pocket that when pressed to the greasy area instantly absorb any excess oils, leaving your face mattified. These can be used as often as you need. Toners are also useful for those with oily skin, removing any impurities and oil residues and helping to close open pores; these can be used several times a day, particularly in hot weather. Common natural astringents that are good for oily skin types are lemon and cucumber. You can mix half a teaspoon of each to apply to your face in the evenings as a natural sebum-clearing remedy. Face masks with a clay base are especially helpful in reducing oil as clay literally soaks up any excess sebum leaving the skin balanced and clear.

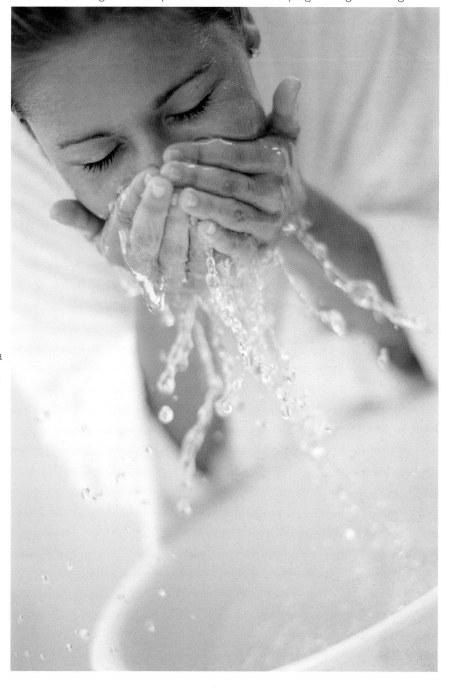

It is important to use a special facial wash if you have oily skin. Your skin needs moisture just the same as everybody else, but you should avoid products that will just make your skin more oily.

Tip 29: *Coping with Acne*

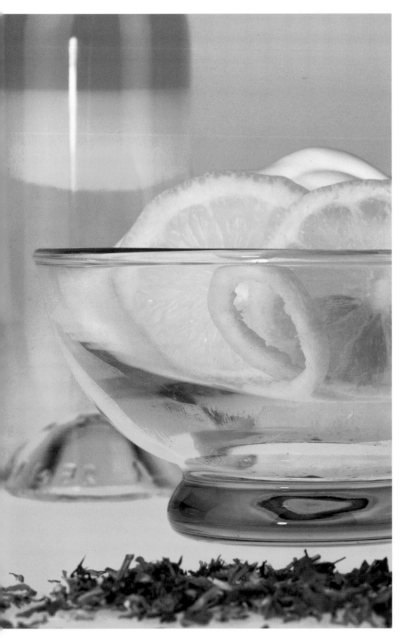

Infusions using comfrey, a medicinal herb that has been used for centuries to treat wounds, can be a very good treatment for acne. The leaves of comfrey contain a substance known as "allantoin," which is responsible for the healing properties of the herb.

Although 80 percent of teenagers suffer from acne, it can strike at any age. Studies have shown that acne in later life can be triggered and exacerbated by problems such as stress, anxiety and depression.

Acne in adolescence is triggered by the male hormone testosterone, which is present in the body to encourage growth. However, it can have an overstimulating effect on the sebaceous glands in the face, leading to blocked pores, blemishes and blackheads. In later life, stress and poor diet are considered aggravating factors in acne, but it is doubtlessly still the excessive sebum that is most to blame.

Anyone with a skin type prone to acne should seek the advice of their doctor. Technological advancements mean that there is plenty of medical help available for this often painful and unsightly condition. These include laser skin treatments and medication. However, if you do decide to treat your acne at home, don't be tempted to pop your pimples as this can lead to both infection and scarring. Wash your face with a mild cleanser morning and night, but don't scrub at your skin – infected and sore complexions should be treated gently. Steer clear of products that contain alcohol as it can make matters worse by encouraging further oil production. The herb comfrey is often found on the ingredient list of natural acne treatments as its skin-healing properties are thought to be helpful for this condition. Consult an herbalist or naturopath who may prescribe a tincture to be applied to outbreaks. Unfortunately, blackheads often accompany acne, and the only way to deal with these blocked pores is to steam them open and, very gently, using a tissue, ease out the plugs of sebum. Cleansing alone will not get rid of blackheads. Once they are out, it is very important to follow a stringent cleansing routine to stop the blackheads from reappearing.

Tip 30: *Caring for Young Skin*

The key to keeping young skin glowing is not to overload it with products, but rather let it breathe naturally. However, it's important to get a cleansing routine established to prevent pores clogging and breakouts occurring. Young skin may benefit from a simple facial wash; choose one that is as natural as possible, and always look for the words "mild" or "gentle." Don't forget any sun damage that occurs will be worn on the face for life, so the sooner sun protection is begun the better for skin health and preventing wrinkles! Drinking plenty of water will also help to keep skin clear, as will a natural and healthy diet that includes plenty of fruits and vegetables. It is also a good idea to cleanse the skin after sports or energetic activities, as sweating opens the pores, which in turn can trap dirt and debris. Look for products that are aimed specifically at young skin, in particular skin milks or light moisturizers that are low on oil in their makeup, or purely natural products that don't contain perfume or chemicals. Any dry patches, on the knees and elbows, for example, can be treated with a natural beeswax or essential-oil-based balm.

Unfortunately, young skin is often problem skin, but blemishes, blackheads and acne can be minimized if you take the right steps. A facial scrub will often remove blackheads, especially if you have opened the pores by steaming your face over a bowl of hot water first. You can help a blemish to dry out more quickly by dabbing it with antiseptic. This is a much better way of dealing with it than squeezing, which can result in bruising and skin damage. Acne is best treated by a visit to your doctor, who, thanks to recent breakthroughs, should be able to prescribe something that can minimize this condition.

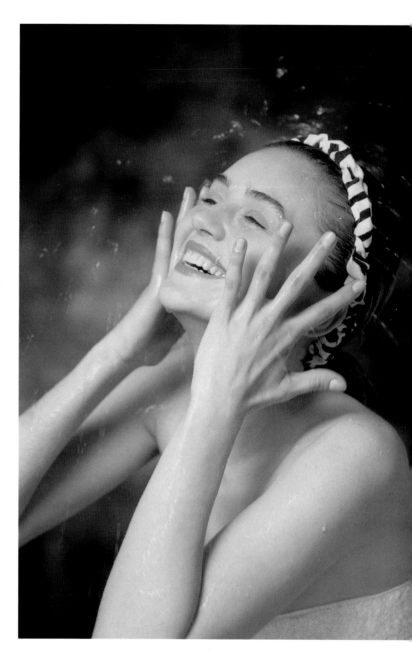

It is important not to overload young skin with too many products. Often, a simple cleansing routine is enough for healthy, glowing skin.

Tip 31: *Caring for Teenage Skin*

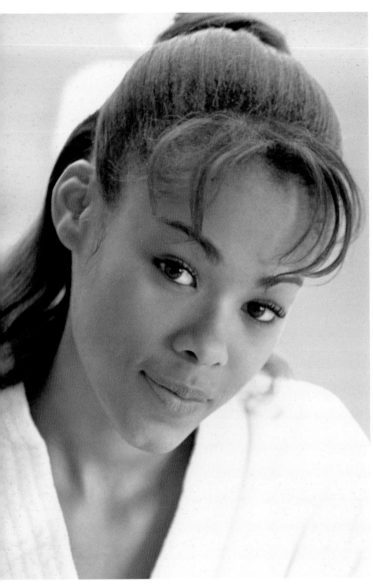

Teenagers often face a multitude of problems with their skin, but steps can be taken to minimize these.

Due to the multitude of hormonal disturbances taking place during puberty, teenage skin is often beset by problems. Blemishes, blackheads and acne are particular problems and can, if serious, affect the confidence and quality of life of a teenager. Coping with the physical and emotional changes of adolescence is difficult enough without the added complication of bad skin. Fortunately, there are a number of ways of minimizing these skin conditions. Blackheads can be removed by using a facial scrub, which is particularly effective if you have helped to open the pores with a steam treatment. Antiseptic can be used to help dry out a blemish. This is a much better way of dealing with spots than squeezing, as this can damage the skin and lead to bruising. Recent breakthroughs in the treatment of acne can offer welcome relief from this distressing condition. Your doctor should be able to prescribe a treatment that will help to minimize outbreaks. In addition to these treatments for skin conditions, drinking plenty of water and maintaining a sensible diet, filled with fresh fruits and vegetables, will certainly help to keep skin clear. Needless to say, keeping junk food and sugary drinks to a minimum will also be of benefit to overall health as well as skin.

Cleansing is an important part of caring for teenage skin. Look for cleansers that are labeled "oil-free," "fragrance-free" and "mild." Anything strong on delicate, teenage skin can cause a reaction, especially as cleansing should be done at least twice a day. A toner is useful for oily teenage skin, but is not essential. Oil-free moisturizers are a great way to keep up skin hydration levels without overloading it with grease, as are oil-free cosmetics, such as mineral powders, which are entirely natural.

The teen years are ideal for getting into a sun-care routine, using sunscreen with a high SPF to avoid skin damage. However, some of these lotions can be too heavy on teenage skin, so look out for sun protection "milk" which is lighter, or natural SPFs in the form of the mineral titanium dioxide.

Tip 32: *Caring for Skin in Your 20s & 30s*

Your 20s are the ideal years to begin a preventative routine that discourages wrinkling and aging in later years. Looking for an antioxidant moisturizer may well prevent many wrinkles from occurring. Even though in the 20s, skin is still considered young, the cell turnover production will have dropped by about 20 percent. Therefore, exfoliating regularly will keep the renewal process going. Cleansing is as important, if not more, than in your teens – makeup removal in particular. Every last trace of make up should be removed in the evenings to prevent pores from clogging. You may wish to invest in a specialized eye makeup remover. These dissolve substances such as mascara much more easily than ordinary skin cleansers, meaning less tugging and pulling around the delicate eye skin.

By the time your 30s arrive, any sun damage you have sustained in your teens and 20s will start to become more obvious, in the form of fine lines and freckles. Expression lines will have begun to appear around your mouth, forehead and eyes, and you may want to adjust your skin care regime to incorporate an antioxidant night cream. A routine that includes AHAs (alpha hydroxy acids) will keep cell renewal at an optimum level, leaving skin looking plumped and more firm. It is important that you continue to protect your skin against the sun, so follow the advice given on page 47.

Of course, it is impossible to turn back the clock and halt the aging process, but you can take steps to prevent skin damage and, by doing so, increase the longevity of healthy, vibrant skin.

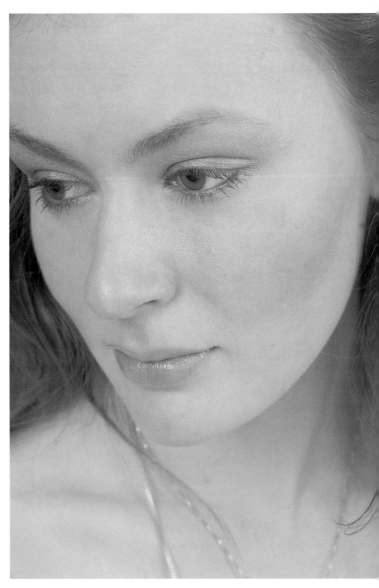

By the time your 30s arrive, any skin damage sustained earlier in life will become noticeable, but it is not too late to prevent further damage.

Tip 33: *Caring for Mature Skin*

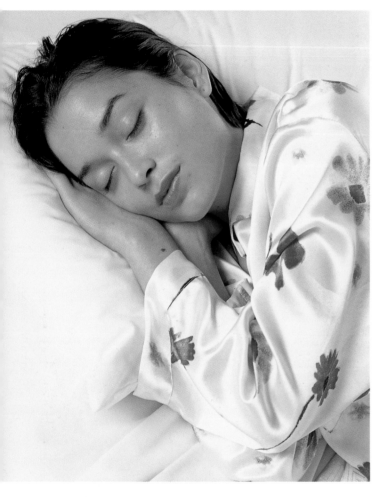

While we are sleeping our bodies are renewing cells, including on the face. Sleep is the cheapest beauty treatment on the planet, and you should try to get your full eight hours!

From the age of 40 and up skin unfortunately begins to lose its elasticity, making the appearance of wrinkles and lines more obvious. Because of the decreasing lack of tone in the depths of the skin, it becomes more difficult for the skin to support itself. Mature skin becomes thinner and more fragile, and requires extra care and support.

While there are many, many creams and potions claiming to reduce wrinkles, it can be baffling when trying to decide what might work. Newer innovations include the addition of calcium to fortify facial and neck skin. Any creams claiming they can reduce lines do so by temporarily plumping the skin, giving a fuller appearance that makes wrinkles less noticeable. Those creams that claim a Botox-like effect to freeze muscles and thereby reduce lines work on a very temporary and surface level. You may be disappointed with the result. Both sun damage and loss of elasticity can give neck skin a loose appearance. While some experts claim that facial exercises can be helpful, many women choose to look for topical support, such as a moisturizer that includes firming abilities.

Certain basics, such as day cream with SPF and a rich night cream, will certainly help the overall effect of your skin, as will exfoliating to uncover newer, plumper skin cells. Smooth, well-hydrated skin automatically looks better and less lined than skin that is dry. As skin matures, incorporating a skin serum into your routine may well pay off in delivering vital antioxidants to protect and nourish. Serums work by placing an intense dose of vitamins directly onto the skin. A once-weekly, deeply hydrating face mask can also give skin more flexibility and the appearance of volume, although this will be temporary.

Even if your skin has sustained sun damage in your earlier years, it is still important to protect both face and neck from the harmful effects of the sun. This will not only prevent further damage being done, but will also reduce your chances of developing skin cancer.

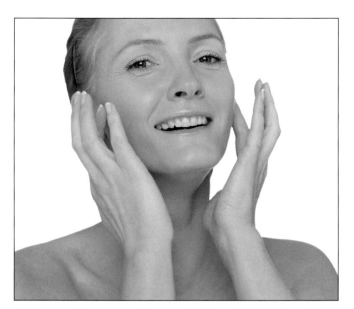

1. One way to increase muscle tone and reduce wrinkling is through invigorating facial massage. Start by gently stroking your face in an upward movement as if you were massaging a smile into place.

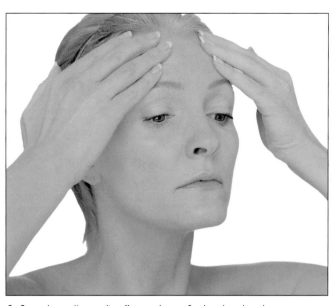

2. Smooth any "worry lines" around your forehead and eyebrows.

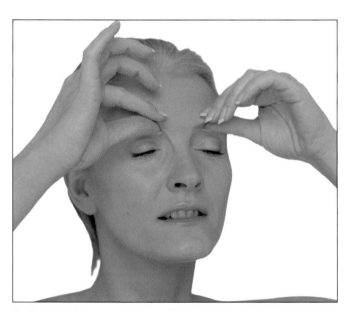

3. Gently pinch your eyebrows to release any pent up tension, then lightly pat your face all over with your fingertips, like raindrops.

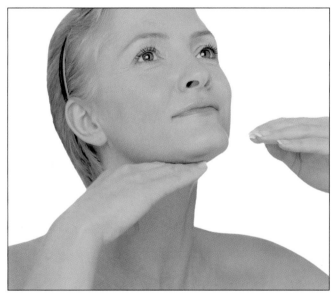

4. Gently pat your chin in an upward direction to encourage firming of the chin and neck muscles.

Sleep is an often overlooked part of a beauty regime, but it is essential if you are to look and feel your best. Sleep is crucial to physical renewal, as the hormones that are necessary for cell growth are inhibited by the hormones that keep us awake. In short, sleep is the time when your body repairs itself, so it is crucial that you get enough of it. Most people need around seven to eight hours a night, but other people need more and some can manage on less. You will know how much you need to feel refreshed and invigorated.

Tip 34: *Wrinkles & Lined Skin*

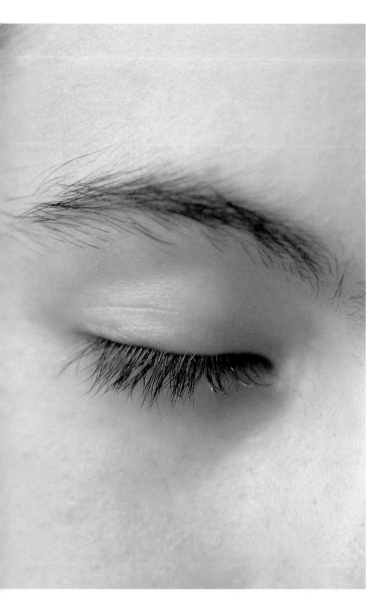

The skin around your eyes is especially prone to wrinkles and crow's-feet. While it is impossible to ward off wrinkles forever, it is possible to reduce the appearance of wrinkles by using a collagen-based moisturizer.

Ultimately, barring a facelift, there is no long-term cure for wrinkles, but many women find collagen moisturizers do help to plump out. Before dismissing lotions and potions entrirely, bear in mind that pharmaceutical companies spend millions on research and production of wrinkle-reducing creams. Some of them work and some of them don't. Always ask for samples first, and try as many as possible to find one that suits your skin. And remember to borrow from friends and relatives – don't feel like you have to buy every product under the sun.

Current trends indicate that many women turn to "fillers" and Botox to reduce the appearance of lines. These treatments, which must be performed by a qualified therapist, certainly do work on reducing wrinkles more dramatically than any creams can, but they are costly and many women don't like the idea of anything invasive. Fillers usually consist of collagen, a substance naturally found in the human body. It is the loss of collagen, which supports the skin, that is the cause of wrinkles. Injectable collagen will temporarily rejuvenate and fill deep lines, sometimes with dramatic effect. Botox, or Botox-like injectables, act to freeze the muscles around wrinkles, so wrinkles reduce because the muscles aren't being used. Neither of these treatments are a pain-free option, as both use needles. Although the therapist gives a localized anesthetic around the area to be treated, it can still be uncomfortable.

Tip 35: *Caring for Your Lips*

Lips need special care as they have no sweat glands and few sebaceous glands, which means that they can dry out very easily.

There are several causes of chapped lips, including dehydration, overexposure to the sun, dry or cold weather and lip biting or sucking. It can also be an indicator that you are lacking in vitamin B2, although in this case, cracks are more likely to occur around the sides or corners of your mouth.

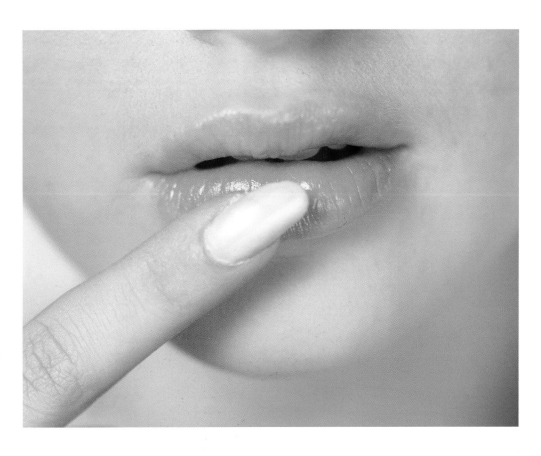

Try not to lick your lips; as saliva dries, it evaporates and has a drying effect. It's a good idea to use lip balm containing vitamin E or pure vitamin E oil to treat lips that have become dry. If lips are flaking, rub a dry washcloth over them very gently to remove any excess skin and follow with a good moisturizer. There are many excellent over-the-counter lip balms available but some contain lanolin, which is a potential allergen, making the condition worse. Many also contain petroleum products and perfumes, which can make lips more sensitive. Natural balms use beeswax or natural oils, such as jojoba or cocoa butter, instead. Whichever one you decide to use, it will act as a barrier between the environment and your lips, keeping them moist and soft. Your lip balm should contain sunscreen to help protect them from the sun's damaging rays. If your lips crack to the extent that they become infected, you should seek advice from your doctor.

Use a lip balm containing vitamin E to keep your lips looking healthy, hydrated and attractive. Alternatively, use pure vitamin E oil.

Tip 36: *Dealing with Cellulite*

Cellulite is caused by deposits of fat underneath the skin's surface, and the common effect is skin dimpling, sometimes known as "orange peel" skin. A large proportion of cellulite is comprised of toxins and fat, and it tends to appear on the butt and thighs, although other common places to find cellulite are the upper arms and stomach. More commonly affecting women than men due to fluctuating hormonal levels, cellulite can be hard to get rid of. A sensible eating plan that is low in fat and high in fiber, and a good, regular exercise program can help to reduce cellulite. Include more fruits and vegetables in your diet. Two-thirds of our diet is often "empty calories": sugars, white flour and processed food. They have little nutritional value, but cause weight gain, as they are stored as fat rather than moving through the digestive system or being burned as energy. For this reason, you do not have to be overweight to have cellulite. Avoiding caffeine, alcohol and sugary foods will help to prevent further cellulite from appearing, and staying properly hydrated by drinking plenty of water can help to disperse toxins.

You can make your own anticellulite treatments. The enzymes and warming stimulation offered by essential oils, kaolin, ginger and strawberries make these ingredients popular.

Many women turn to products to give skin a smoother appearance. In fact, it is most likely to be the massaging action in applying the creams that is of the most benefit, but some do increase circulation, which in turn will help the overall appearance of any lumps and bumps. Salon treatments are available to treat cellulite – usually an intensive course of either therapist- or machine-based massage – but these can be expensive.

Tip 37: *Dealing with Stretch Marks*

Stretch marks are easily recognizable by their almost silvery appearance where skin has been stretched. Stretch marks begin with a reddish color, often turning to a deep purple, and eventually fade out to a lighter shade than your natural skin tone, making them more noticeable. Beginning in the middle layers of the skin, stretch marks occur when skin is stretched over a period of time, causing a loss of elasticity and the breakage of small connective fibers. The most common causes of stretch marks are weight gain, rapid weight loss and pregnancy, when the skin, particularly over the stomach and breasts, is stretched to its limits. Unfortunately, little can be done to minimize stretch marks, and even less to get rid of them completely. Many women find massaging their stomachs and thighs with vitamin E oil can help to prevent stretch marks occurring during pregnancy by giving the skin more elasticity. Cocoa butter and shea butter also work well as intensive moisturizing treatments for stretched skin. Both men and women can experience stretch marks, particularly those whose weight fluctuates: for example body builders and athletes are prone to stretch marks.

Stretch marks are more noticable on paler skins tones, so if you have this type of skin a good way of disguising stretch marks is to use fake tan solutions, which help to reduce their appearance.

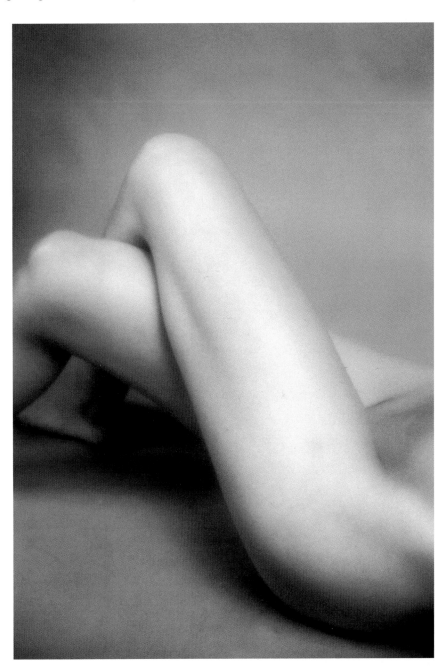

Stretch marks are particularly prevalent on the thighs and the stomach. If you have pale skin, as good way of disguising them is to use fake tan solutions.

Tip 38: *Beautiful Hands*

Hands are regularly exposed to extreme conditions, so it is important to look after them if their skin is to remain soft and supple. Although many of us neglect our hands, they can respond beautifully to intense bursts of treatment. There are few oil glands on the backs of our hands, which is why they can wrinkle so quickly, plus factor in the number of times hands are immersed in soap and water, and it's easy to see why they can look uncared for. Also, it is important to bear in mind that hands are exposed virtually all the time, so they are as prone to environmental and sun damage as your face. Regular exfoliation of the hands gives a good result and kickstarts the cell renewal process to reveal younger cells underneath. Follow exfoliation with a rich hand or body cream and rub in liberally. It is also a wise idea to use sunscreen on your hands every single day to shield them from further sun damage. After every water immersion, always rub cream into your hands, and when possible, use rubber gloves to keep them completely dry. Regular manicures will make your hands look well groomed and fresh.

The two most common hand problems are dry skin and brittle nails, so give yourself a manicure once a week and finish with a deep-moisturizing treatment for both hands and nails.

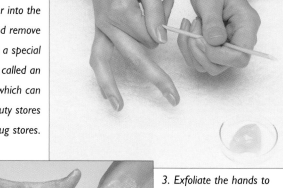

1. Wash your hands with a gentle soap and then immerse them in a bowl of warm water containing one drop of chamomile essential oil. Leave to soak for five minutes.

2. Dry your hands, then rub cuticle remover into the nail bases and remove cuticles with a special implement called an "orange stick," which can be bought in beauty stores and some drug stores.

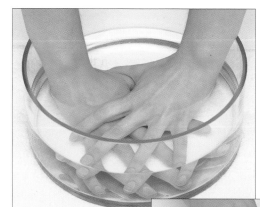

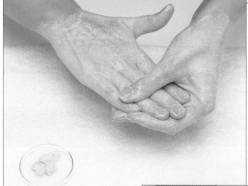

3. Exfoliate the hands to remove dead skin cells, then liberally apply rich hand or body cream to help rehydrate the skin.

4. Apply nail polish if desired; use a base coat to avoid staining.

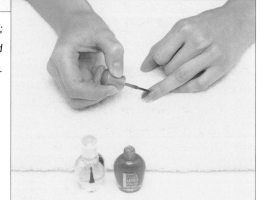

Tip 39: *Attractive, Healthy Feet*

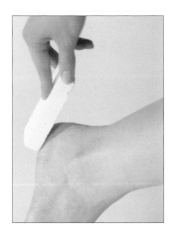

1. Wash each foot in warm water, then gently rub the soles and heels with a pumice stone to remove hard skin.

2. Dry the feet thoroughly, especially between the toes.

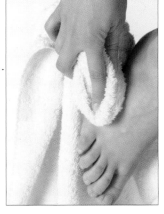

3. Trim the nails with nail clippers or scissors, cutting them straight across. Do not cut down the sides of the nails, as this can increase your chances of getting ingrown toenails.

Feet need special attention, not only to look as pretty as possible, but also to function well. You will walk about 70,000 miles (110,000 km) miles in your lifetime — that's four times around the world — so regular care of your feet is a worthwhile investment.

A common problem with feet is dry skin and heel cracking, which can be painful and unsightly. Dry feet lack moisture, but where sections of hard skin build up can be due to inappropriate footwear, such as strappy shoes. Patches of hard skin should be filed away and then liberally moisturized, as should cracked heels. If the problem is excessive or you are unable to easily get rid of hardened areas you should consult a podiatrist, or foot care expert. Feet that are dry and flaky, however, can be exfoliated the same as any other part of your body, followed by applying a moisturizer or intensive oil. Regular nail clipping and filing is essential to a well-groomed look for feet and this should be done by cutting in a straight line across the top of the nail — never from inner to outer corner as this is believed to cause ingrown toenails.

4. Rub petroleum jelly or cuticle cream into the sides and base of the nails with your fingertips, then with the blunt end of a special implement called an "orange stick," work at the sides and base of the nails to ease the skin back.

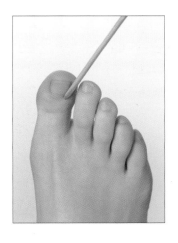

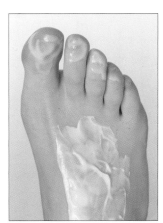

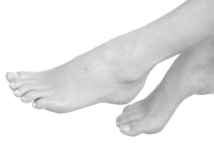

5. Rub the feet and nails all over with cream specially designed for the feet, or with hand or body cream.

Tip 40: *Caring for the Eye Area*

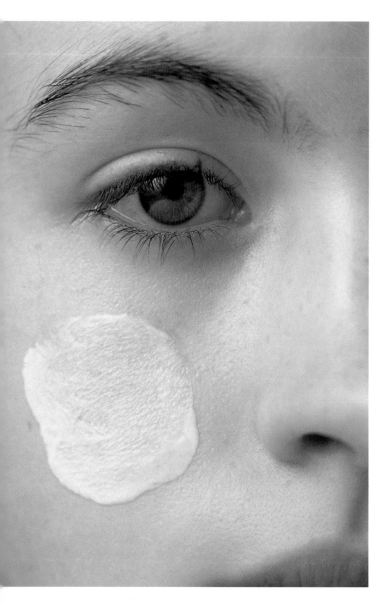

Moisturize the area around the eye very carefully, as the skin there is very delicate and can be easily damaged. Your regular moisturizer should be fine for the skin around your eyes, and there probably isn't any need for a separate moisturizer for the eye area.

Our eyes make more than 100,000 movements a day, so they deserve attention from time to time. We often neglect our eyes without realizing it, by exposing them to smoky environments or by not removing eye makeup. Eyes often become tired and sore after a day spent in front of a computer screen or reading small print. Always make sure that you work in well-lit conditions, and if you suffer from eyestrain, have your eyes tested regularly.

The skin around our eyes is extremely delicate and you should never, tug, pull or rub it as this will lead to premature wrinkling. Treat it as you would treat tissue paper – with gentleness and care. Although there are many products that promise to banish undereye bags and dark circles, these can be limited in their success. Usually undereye bags are due to swelling – possibly caused by crying, fluid retention or hay fever – and anything cooling will help to reduce this. Sliced cucumber from the fridge is a favorite, although it is probably the cooling action rather than the cucumber that has the effect! The application of moisturizer around the eye area should be done delicately – dab some cream above and around the outer eye corner and gently pat over the whole eye area without rubbing. Products for dark circles rarely reduce this often genetic problem, but concealers with light-reflecting particles reduce the shading significantly by bouncing light away from the dark areas. The jury is still out on whether separate moisturizers for the eye area are necessary and you will find as many experts who say it is essential as those who will say it isn't! Moisturizers and wrinkle-reducing creams tend to be of a lighter consistency than those designed for the rest of the face which is likely to help absorption. A worthwhile investment, however, is a special eye makeup remover, as these dissolve mascara and eyeliner more easily, which means less rubbing to remove makeup. In the long term, this could mean fewer wrinkles!

Like any other part of the body, eyes respond well to drinking plenty of water, a healthy diet rich in fruits and vegetables, and getting a good enough amount of sleep. Your overall health is reflected in your eyes – eyes that are clear and sparkling always look beautiful. If you detect any redness or itchiness in and around your eyes, you should always consult your doctor, as this could be due to a makeup allergy, hay fever or a mild eye infection. To protect your eyes from infections be extra vigilant about cleaning your makeup tools with a mild detergent, and dispose of old mascaras and eyeliners regularly. It is thought that pumping your mascara wand in and out of the jar allows air into the product, which can lead to contamination.

For a cheap but effective treatment for tired eyes, immerse two teabags in hot water, squeeze out the excess moisture, and, when cool, place them over your closed eyes for a few minutes. Tea is mildly astringent and will cool and relax the eyes. Next, place a cucumber slice over each eye. Lie back and let the cooling cucumber do its work. Remove, rinse your eyes with cold water and pat dry.

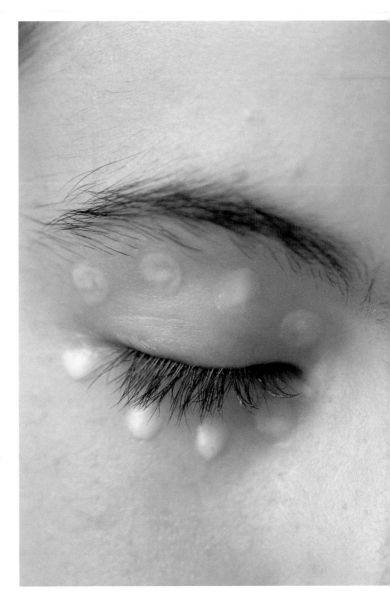

You can reduce the appearance of swelling and bags under the eyes with anything cool. A cheap but effective treatment is a slice of refrigerated cucumber. Products that claim to treat bags under the eyes are not likely to be effective.

Tip 41: *Moisturizing Your Body*

The skin on your body needs just as much care as on your face, and responds well to pampering. Dry skin on the body can feel uncomfortably tight – itchy even – so keeping it well conditioned will not only help the overall look, but the health as well. Exfoliate using buffing grains, salt scrubs or a loofah to buff away dead skin cells. Pay particular attention to your lower legs, which are prone to dryness as the skin is thinner on the front calves. Whether you prefer oil or a lotion, you should add moisture every time you bathe, shower or exfoliate, and regular moisturizing will pay off in the form of softer and smoother skin. As your skin's needs change throughout the year, you may want to swap a heavy duty moisturizer for a lighter one during the summer months. Either way look for oils that absorb quickly and easily, and allow a little time for proper absorption before getting dressed. Even pure olive oil will tackle dry skin, although you may not like the unadulterated smell, which can be strong. Brands that use natural oils are more likely to be in tune with your skin, and are a great way to add a natural fragrance. Popular and effective moisturizers include jojoba, olive oil, vitamin E–rich oil and evening primrose oil.

A good way to restore moisture to the skin on your body is to add a few drops of oil to your bath water. Do not add more than 2 teaspoons (10 ml) or your skin will become too greasy. Always use oils that are appropriate to your skin type. For dry skin, use avocado, wheat-germ, castor or sesame oil; for normal skin, use almond, apricot, jojoba or vitamin E rich oil; and for oily skin, use safflower, camelia or calendula oil.

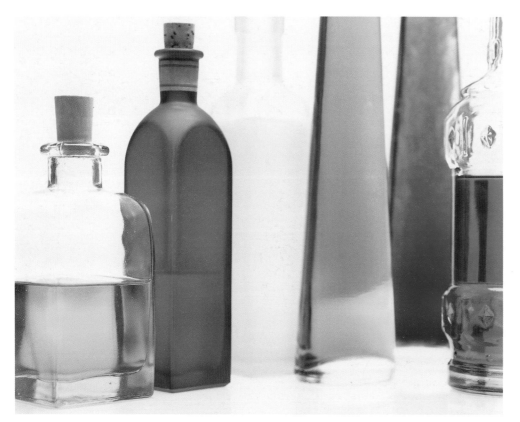

Popular and effective moisturizers include jojoba, olive oil, vitamin E oil and evening primrose oil. When using oils, ensure you pick suitable ones for your skin type.

Tip 42: *Deep Cleansing*

Although it is tempting to go overboard in deep cleansing your face, make it a once a week routine. Any more can cause the skin to become oversensitive. The aim of a deep cleanse is to reach more impurities than normal cleansing on a daily basis can do. There are plenty of deep cleansing masks, usually containing clay to help draw out blackheads, and while they can be very effective, a cheaper home option is to gently steam your face over a bowl of hot water. As the skin warms, the pores open, and you will be able to extract any deeply imbedded impurities. Add essential oils to the steam to make it a relaxing inhalation experience as well. Don't squeeze at anything that is reluctant to come out! This can lead to infection. A deep cleansing salon treatment with a qualified therapist will be able to get rid of deeply imbedded blackheads. Cleansing oils are just as effective as lotion or cream cleansers – in fact, if your skin is dry, you may find oils more gentle and effective. Using small circular motions all over your face, gently rub in the oil and wipe away with a tissue. Using a massage action with a facial oil is more beneficial that simply swiping with cotton pads and can give a deeper clean.

You can take cleansing treatments a stage further if you wish and visit a sauna. Sweating it out in the sauna is one of the simplest and most effective ways to cleanse your body from within. Carrying impurities out of your system by natural means, a sauna has benefits for your health, appearance and well-being. A good time to take a sauna is after exercise, as the heat can flush out lactic acid from your muscles. Remember to take a cool shower after a sauna and drink lots of water.

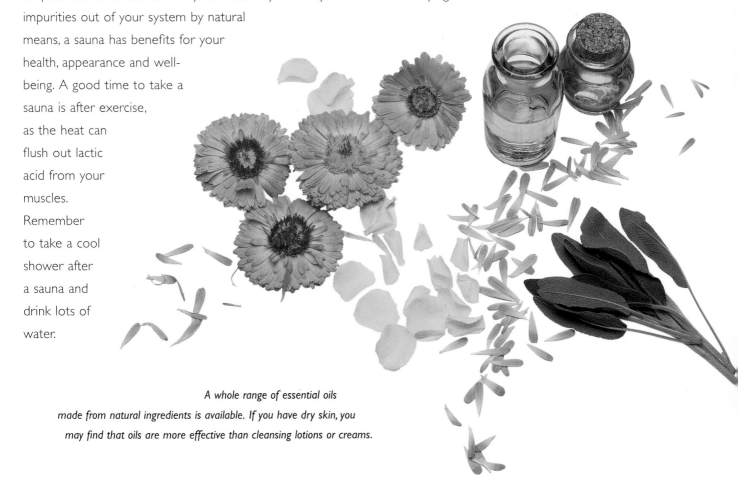

A whole range of essential oils made from natural ingredients is available. If you have dry skin, you may find that oils are more effective than cleansing lotions or creams.

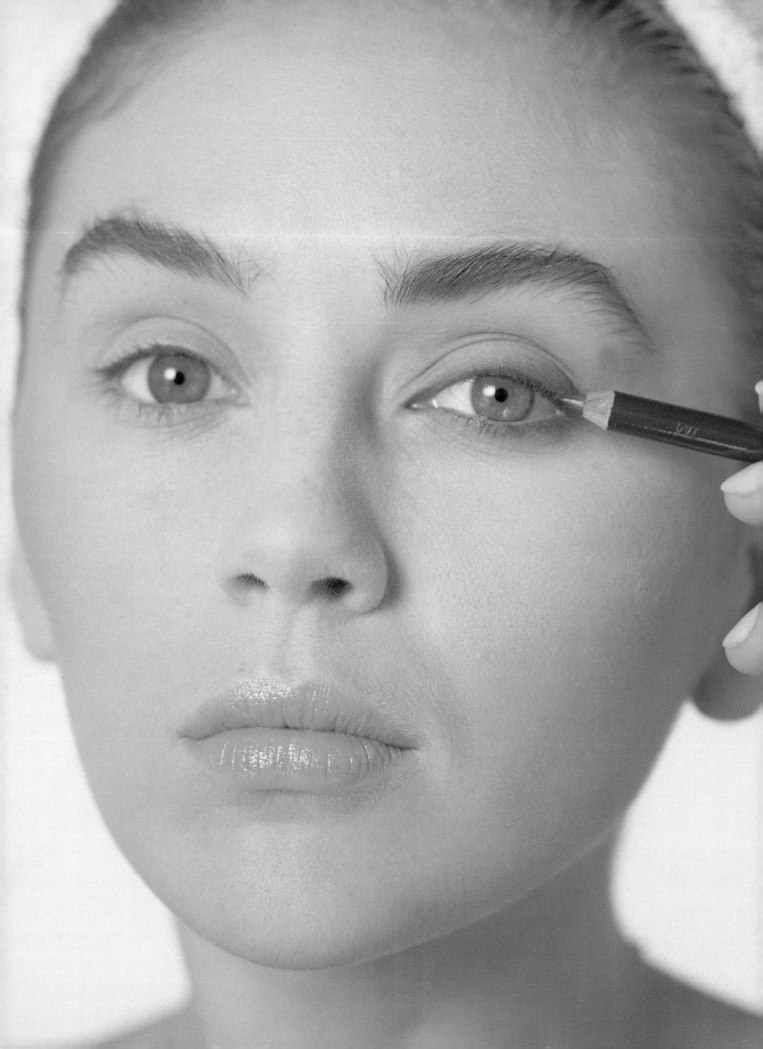

chapter three
EYES AND MAKEUP

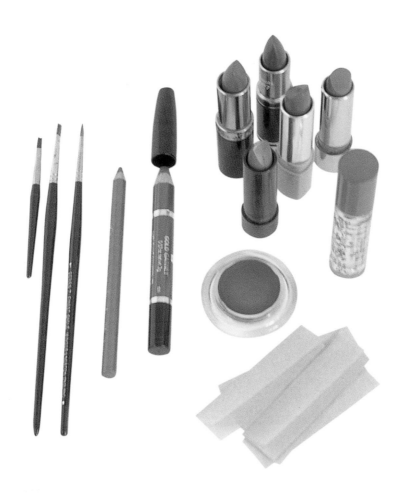

Tip 43: *Preparing Your Face for Makeup*

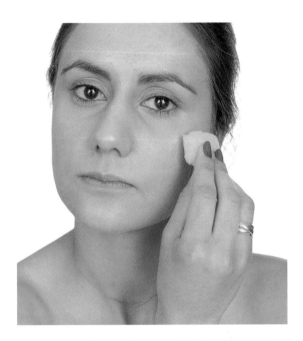

It is important that you cleanse your face thoroughly before applying makeup. Use a cleansing cream or lotion, or if you have dry skin, you may prefer to use a cleansing oil.

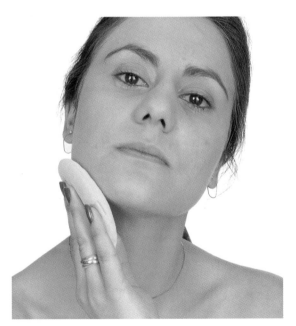

When cleansing, ensure you do a thorough job and cover your entire face. Once you have cleansed and rinsed your face, apply moisturizer.

No professional makeup artist will ever begin to apply makeup until the model's face has been thoroughly cleansed and moisturized. Makeup applied to skin that is not scrupulously clean will clog the pores and skin will look stale and unattractive. Moisturizers are important for nourishing and protecting the skin. They leave it soft and smooth so that foundation can be applied evenly. Allow your moisturizer a little time to sink in before you begin to apply foundation. Most makeup artists will use a primer before applying any cosmetics. Primers act as a skin smoother, allowing foundation to be applied with more fluidity and give better, more even results. It allows foundation to "glide" across the skin, rather than having to be worked in. In truth, unless you are a catwalk star, primers aren't necessary, but more an added extra. You can get a similar priming effect from moisturizing effectively and ensuring that you have given it adequate time – usually about 10 minutes – to sink into your skin properly. If you are going to apply evening makeup, look for a moisturizing and firming face mask to use beforehand. You are unlikely to need a moisturizer on top of this unless your skin is very dry. Use a specialized, oil-based eye makeup remover to properly dissolve any left over mascara or liner around the eyes, and don't forget your eyebrows! Brows also need cleaning but are often forgotten – dry skin under the hairs can become flaky and obvious, and any residues of brow liner or gel can quickly build up to become clumpy.

Tip 44: *Makeup Removal*

Always, always remove your makeup before you go to bed at night! Leaving your makeup on can lead to eye infections and breakouts because your skin can't breathe correctly. At night, skin goes through a natural regeneration process, so unremoved makeup can disrupt this. The best way to remove makeup is by using a cleanser, which helps loosen the makeup from your face and will leave your skin feeling fresh and able to breathe. Cleansers come in various consistencies – you may prefer a facial wash, to be used with warm water, and a washcloth. These are good for oily skin but don't always deliver on removing eye makeup. A cleansing milk is a light, cream formula, great for young skin and should be applied to the face like a moisturizer and then gently tissued off or swept away with a cotton pad. Cleansing creams or balms have a thicker consistency, and are good for drier skin types. They are also better at dissolving eye makeup, although a specialized eye makeup remover is best to avoid stinging. Always treat the area around the eyes with great care when cleansing, as the skin tissue in this area is particularly sensitive. Avoid stretching and harsh rubbing of the skin, which could result in irritation and swelling. To apply eye makeup remover, simply dab the liquid or cream onto a cotton ball and gently wipe around the eye area. Don't apply it directly to your eye and then remove it, as you will end up with greasy, sticky eyes.

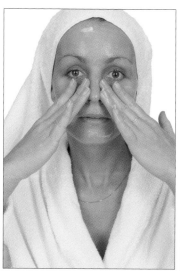

1. Choose a light cream or liquid cleanser that suits your skin and spread it all over your face and neck.

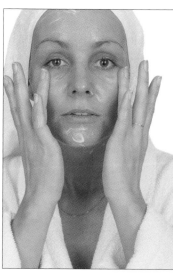

2. Rub the cleanser well into your face but try not to drag the skin. Smooth it in with your fingertips, always using upward movements.

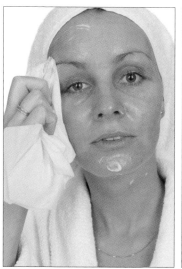

3. To remove the cleanser, gently wipe your face with a paper tissue, taking care not to rub your skin too harshly.

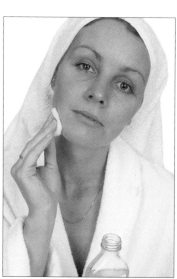

4. Splash your face with cold water to remove the cleanser and makeup.

Tip 45: *Choosing Makeup for Your Skin Type*

No two people have identical skin. In addition, the condition of your skin can vary from week to week and day to day, depending on the weather, your diet, your emotional state and your general health. Picking the right makeup for your skin type can prevent further problems and make the most of your complexion.

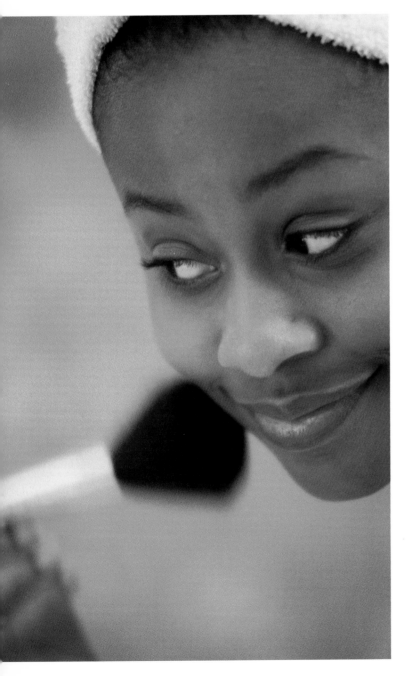

Oily Skin

Choose oil-free foundations that won't compound your oil problem or block pores. Although there are many types of blush and eye shadows, avoid those that have a creamy consistency as they contain far more oil than others. Add them to oily skin and not only will they literally slide off your face as the day goes on, but they can cause pores to block and more blemishes to occur. Stick to powder, which won't crease or smudge on oil-prone skin. If you have oily skin, it is particularly important that you follow a thorough, but gentle cleansing routine, removing all traces of grease, grime and makeup each night to prevent clogged-up pores erupting into unsightly blemishes and blackheads.

Dry Skin

The opposite of oily skin, you are looking for a foundation that also adds moisture to your skin to prevent your "base" from looking caked or cracked. The same applies to eye shadows – always opt for cream shadows, or if you use powdery ones, make sure that your skin is well moisturized underneath. Eye makeup tends to "disappear" on dry lids; try an eye shadow primer to help the color particles adhere for longer.

If you have oily skin, ensure your makeup doesn't have a creamy consistency, as this will only add to the problem.

Combination Skin

It may be beneficial for combination skin types to wear two different textures of foundation on the skin, but ensuring the same color. For the oily T-zone, an oil-free foundation will work to keep your skin looking matte and composed, while a moisturizing foundation will tackle any dryness in the surrounding areas. Depending upon where your oil flare-ups occur, cream-to-powder eye shadows can work well, being neither too oily nor too dry. As with oily skin, it is essential for combination skin to be treated with careful and methodical cleansing before applying makeup and when removing it.

Normal Skin

Normal skin types should stick to a lightly moisturizing foundation, but are lucky enough to take their pick when it comes to blush and eye shadows. You may find your skin varies from time to time in its level of dryness, so have a selection of cream and powder shades to play with.

Blemished Skin

Experts would say that if you have problem skin you shouldn't wear makeup at all, however it is people with this skin type whose confidence is boosted most by coverage. Look for mineral foundations – literally ground minerals, both pure and natural, that allow the skin to breathe and give coverage. Some skin experts claim mineral makeup can help to treat acne and scarring thanks to its anti-inflammatory properties, and because inert minerals are unable to support bacteria. It also carries a natural SPF of between 15 and 20.

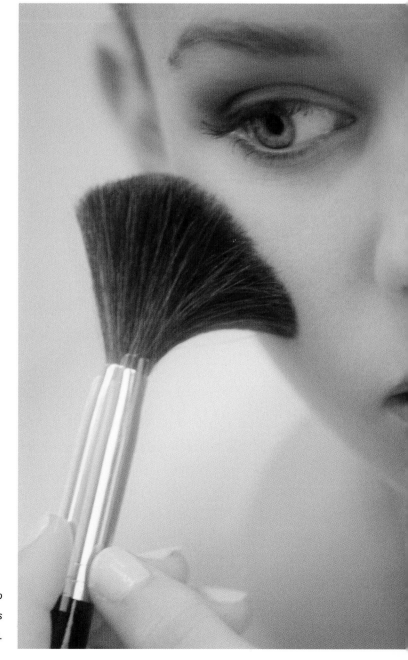

Those of you lucky enough to have a normal skin type are free to choose a variety of products. It is a good idea to have both creams and powders available for when the dryness of your skin varies.

Tip 46: *Choosing Makeup for Your Skin Tone and Eye Color*

Black Skin Tones

Black skin varies in tone, and one of the most effective ways to "lift" the skin tone is to steer clear of pale, ashy colors, such as light pink, peach or taupe. Makeup with deep pigments work best for darker skin, complementing the skin's natural tones. Opt for caramels, soft browns, golds and deep greens around the eyes, while lips can carry richer, more dramatic shades. The darker your skin tone, usually the darker your lips, so try berry or wine colors such as burgundies or deep reds. Dark skin tones suit blush that isn't too obvious; well-blended, creamy shades of dark pinks and plums, and nonshimmering bronzes give a healthy glow.

White Skin Tones

The paler your skin tone, the more obvious bright colors will look, so when choosing shades, remember the "less is more" principle. Pinks are a safe bet as they suit everyone, and can open up the eyes, giving a "wide awake" look. Blue and green eyes are always enhanced by eyeliners, but steer clear of deep black liners around light eyes. Instead, look for navy, violets, smoky greens and grays. Tawny or pink blush looks more natural than brick-orange or browns. Redheads tend to have very pale skin, and often think they can't wear pinks, instead opting for oranges and corals. However, pink cheeks give a flush of healthy color for a lifted and more vibrant appearance.

Asian Skin Tones (Far East)

Makeup artists will always use cosmetics that have a yellow base on Asian skin to even out imperfections and brighten the tone. This skin tone is best suited to tawny or spicy shades for a more natural look. Browns, apricots, plums and coppers all enliven the face, while opting for reds and browns on lips will complement your natural coloring. Eyeliners can be dark for a smoky effect; try dark brown instead of black, and if your skin tone is light, try pink lips. However, well-blended turquoise greens, bright pinks and even yellows can make the eyes look stunning for the more adventurous.

Asian Skin Tones (India and Pakistan sub-continent)

Your skin tone is perfect for yellow-based foundations, and deep, rich, jewel eye shadows. Soft tones can look also look beautiful; greens, hazels and deep pinks are all natural accompaniments to this tone. Steer clear of oranges and corals, or overly pale shades. Carefully blended eyeliner can give eyes a vibrant, smoky look; forest green looks stunning, as does copper. Pale lipsticks will give a washed-out effect to the face and should be avoided; rich reds and lush browns are more complimentary and enlivening.

Tip 47: *Your Makeup Bag Essentials*

Most makeup bags are a mishmash of old favorites and one or two never-wear mistakes. However, updating and refreshing your look largely depends upon how well your basics are chosen. Many women are reluctant to spend money on makeup tools, but these can make or break your makeup application, and are as important as your cosmetics to get a refined and foolproof look. Most makeup now has a best-before date, so don't hang on to old products that won't do their job properly anymore. Anything that looks or smells "odd" should be thrown away immediately as the contents have deteriorated. Look for a box with drawers to keep everything on hand and organized.

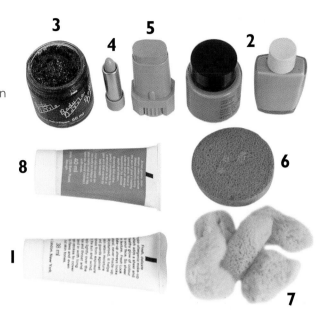

Foundation

Your foundation is designed to even out your skin tone, rather than give color. A perfectly matched foundation is the canvas for the rest of your makeup. Cream (1) and liquid (2) foundations are available.

Blush

It's a good idea to have at least two or three blushes (9) in your basic makeup kit. At least one should be a neutral, cream blush for daytime wear, while the others can be more lively shades for evenings and dramatic makeup looks.

Concealer

Every makeup bag should contain at least a couple of concealers. A green-based one will neutralize redness, while light reflective concealers bounce away dark undereye circles. A concealer stick (4) will cover blemishes and an olive pan-stick (5) will help to mask shadows.

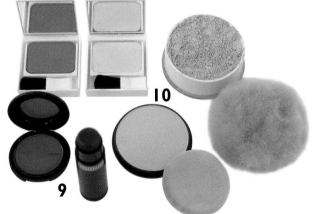

Sponge Applicator

While many women are happy just using their fingers to blend in their base, using a wedge-shaped, soft sponge or latex applicator will give a better, more even finish. These can be bought in packs at any drug store. Keep them scrupulously clean by washing in mild soap, or simply throw away after a week. Synthetic (6) and natural sea sponges (7) are available.

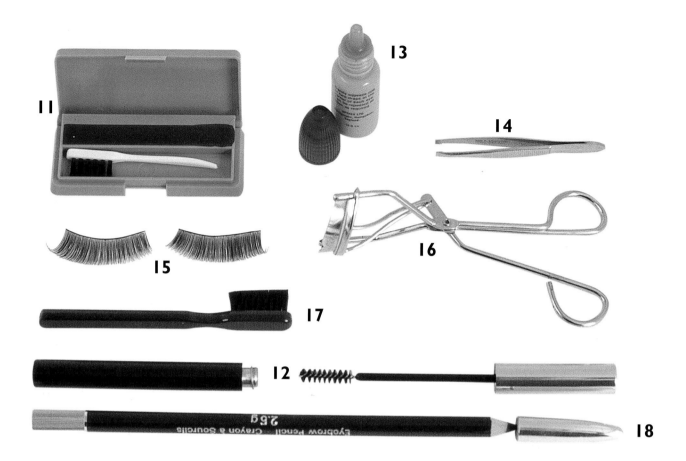

Blush Brush

A soft, fat blush brush gives a pop of color to the cheeks in a very natural-looking way that is hard to replicate with fingers. It can also be used to sweep powder over the face, but ensure you have tapped away any residual blush first.

Powder

Face powder (10) is available in a wide range of shades and textures. However, a light, translucent powder, applied sparingly just to give a matte finish and prevent your foundation from streaking or running, is usually all that is required for a fresh "unclogged" look.

Tinted Moisturizer

Part hydrating treatment, part cosmetic, a tinted moisturizer (8) is perfect for a natural, luminous look. Lighter than full foundation, it gently tints the skin and moisturizes at the same time. Perfect for hot days or when skin is dry and dull.

Eye Shadow Palette

The joy of a color palette (26) is that it stops your makeup bag from getting filled up with lots of separate little single-color containers. A well-chosen palette gives you a choice of colors to work with. Look out for refillable palettes so if one shade is used more than the others you can top it up. Eye shadow pencils (28), liquid eye shadows (31) and cream shadows (32) are also available.

Mascara

Two mascaras: one black and one brown, and preferably waterproof for daytime or evening lashes. Block mascaras (11) and liquid wand mascaras (12) are available.

Eyeliner

Eyeliners give the eyes definition. Depending upon your choice of eyeshadow palette, a coordinating liner will liven up your eyes. Kohl eyeliners (27) will give a bold look.

Lip Balm

A lip balm (23) is probably the most versatile item in your makeup bag! It can be used to soothe chapped lips, smooth unruly eyebrows or give sheen highlighting to the cheeks.

Lip Gloss

A range of lip glosses (24) in your favorite shades give versatility and flexibility to your look. Pick two or three to have as staples.

Lipstick

More matte in consistency than glosses, lipsticks (22) have more staying power and color pigmentation. If you have a lip color you love, buy more than one as lipsticks have a habit of being discontinued!

Eye Shadow Brush

An eye shadow brush (30) should be blunt at the tip, soft and full. This helps with blending and even application. Choose natural fibers where possible.

Other Equipment

A mid-brown brow liner will define your brows and help you create a perfect arch. Sparkling body gel (3) may be used on your face, but not around the eyes. Block mascara (11) must be dampened before use. Eyedrops (13) can be used to make eyes sparkle. Tweezers (14) are useful for plucking eyebrows. False eyelashes (15) are fun accessories. Eyelash curlers (16) can create beautifully upturned lashes. A small brush (17) can be used to style eyebrows, and an eyebrow pencil will be needed if you need to draw these on. Lip brushes (19) can be used for more intricate application of color than a lipstick. A thin lip pencil (20) is used for outlining and a thick lip pencil (21) for filling in. Tissues (25) are useful for blotting.

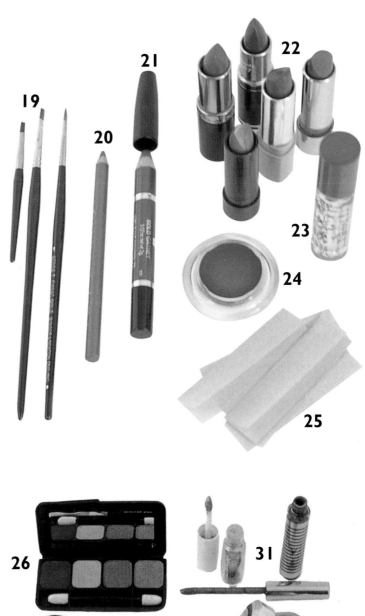

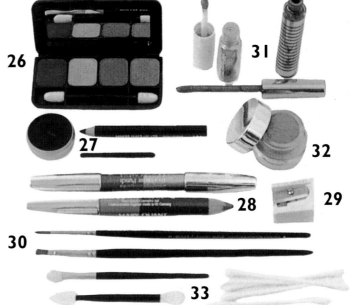

Tip 48: *Looking After Your Makeup*

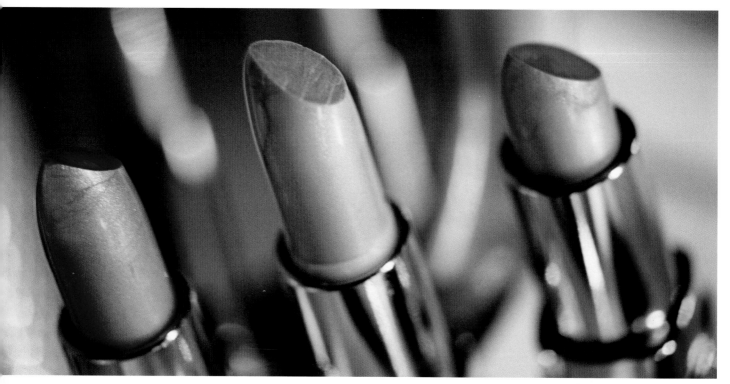

Don't forget that makeup, just like food, will only keep for so long. Once your makeup is beyond a certain age, it should be thrown away and replaced.

Makeup does deteriorate, so stick rigidly to the best-before dates, or make a note of how long they last. As a general rule, foundations, powders, eye shadows, blushes and moisturizers will stay good for 12 to 18 months, and lipsticks for a year. Eyeliners and mascaras should be regularly replaced every 3 months to avoid infections. After a few months, it is advisable to wipe down your makeup compacts and exteriors with a mild soap to keep any germs at bay, and don't forget to wash out your bag or box by wiping with a clean cloth. Makeup that has deteriorated often goes pale or changes consistency – possibly pooling oil – and can even start to smell "off" or musty. Throw any items like this away. To minimize the risk of eye infections and cold sores, don't share your makeup with others. A good point to remember on hygiene is don't ever swipe your lips with the sample lipsticks or glosses at the department store counters – you don't know who you are sharing germs with! Makeup tools also need care; there are brush washes available on the market, but once again, a mild soap-based cleaner (such as dishwashing liquid) will be adequate. Dry your brushes by patting them between two sections of towel and leaving them to air dry before fluffing up. Never leave your makeup near a radiator or in direct sunlight as this will cause them to melt and lose their consistency.

A lot of the time, looking after your makeup is just common sense. You follow basic hygiene rules when preparing food, so approach your makeup in a similar way. There is no point in taking any risks with your health, so if you are in any doubt about your makeup, it is advisable to throw it away, buy some more and make an effort to look after it and keep track of its age.

Tip 49: *Applying Makeup for Your Face Shape*

Not everyone can be an outstanding beauty but, equally, no one is really ever "plain" or "ordinary." Many of the world's most admired models, actresses and celebrities might still be languishing under the label of "Plain Jane" if they had not learned how to make the most of their looks.

Cosmetics have a vital part to play in enhancing and bringing out your features to make you look your best. As a first step to identifying your good points – as well as coping with those that are not as satisfactory – study your face carefully in a mirror. Although every face is unique, most will fall into one of the following categories. By determining your face shape you can learn where the emphasis on your makeup should be to make the most of your assets and hide any imperfections. Shading with foundation, however, is complicated and unless you take a professional makeup artist lesson, hard to achieve.

Oval Face

You have a square chin with a wide, high forehead and the sides of your face are flat. Blush can be applied to the "apples" of the cheeks to give a rounder effect.

Round Face

With full cheeks, your face is a symmetrical and uniform size, with no jutting or angular features. Applying blush just under the cheek bones will give a narrowing effect. You can also apply a light foundation shade over the center of your nose to narrow.

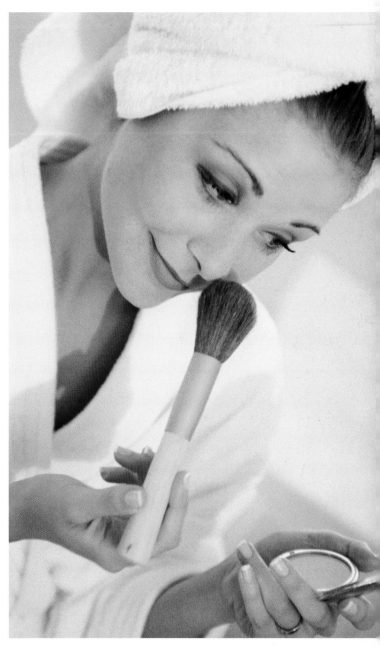

An oval face can benefit from some blush added to the "apples" of the cheeks.

Heart-shaped Face

Wider at the forehead and narrowing toward the chin, a heart-shaped face should use blush on the cheekbones, blending carefully and avoiding the center of the face. This gives a balancing effect.

Long Face

Your features are long and angular with most of the length being from the eye to the chin area. Blush on the cheekbones and blended toward the cheek apples will shorten the area. You can also get a shortening effect from applying highlighter to the chin.

Deep-set Eyes

Avoid dark colors and apply highlighter to the brow bone to bring the eyes "forward." Steer clear of lining the inner rim of the eyes as these will make them seem more recessed.

Close-set Eyes

In order to make eyes appear further apart, use a darker shade eye shadow on the lids from the far corner and blend to the middle of the eye and no further. Put emphasis on the outer lashes when applying mascara.

Narrow/Small Eyes

Your eyes will appear wider if you stick to lighter shades: pearls, pinks and neutrals to open up the eye. Line underneath the eye, but only in the outer corners with a soft pencil. Mascaras that lift the lashes are also "opening."

Wide-set Eyes

Blend a darker color on the eyelid before the crease of your eye, and fade out with a lighter shade to the corner. This color shading brings eyes closer together. Ensure that the fine lashes in the inner eye corners get full coverage with mascara.

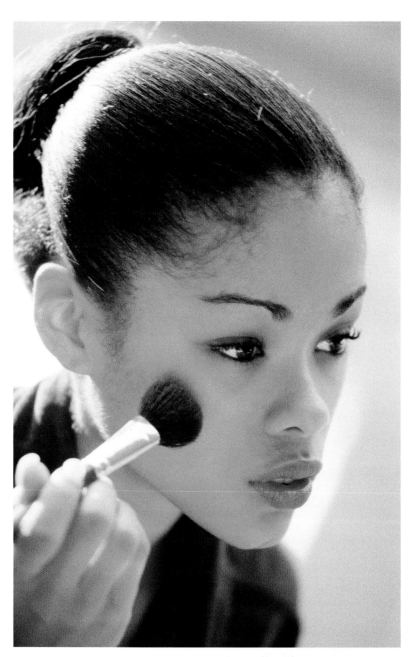

Applying blush just below the cheekbones will help to give a narrowing effect to a round face.

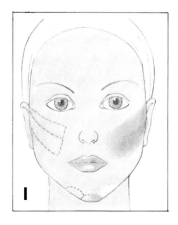

1

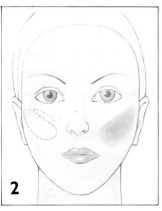

2

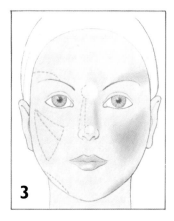

3

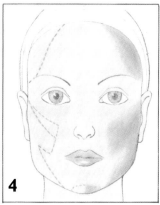

4

To bring out the best in a heart-shaped face, highlight the cheekbones with white. Put blusher beneath this and on the chin.

Emphasize the excellent structure of an oval face with gentle shading on the cheekbones to make them more pronounced.

Thin a round face by shading the jaw line, the cheeks and above the brow bone. Also, highlight the sides and tip of the nose.

Soften a square face with shading from the jaw line to the cheeks. Then narrow the face with color above the temples.

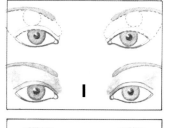

1

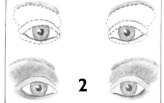

2

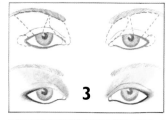

3

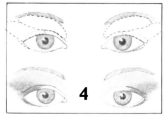

4

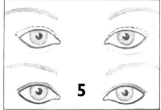

5

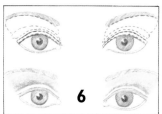

6

In these diagrams eyes without makeup are given above with the corrected eyes underneath. To improve your eyes, apply makeup as indicated by the dotted lines. Wide-set eyes (1) will appear closer together by drawing a bright line inside the lower lashes and by highlighting the center of the lid. Never outline small eyes (2) but use a light shadow on the lid. Make sleepy eyes (3) look more awake with a line above the upper lashes and pale shadow on the lid. For eyes that are set too close together (4) put pale colors on the inner half of the lid, and darker on the outer. Improve protruding eyes (5) with plenty of dark eyeliner. On deep-set eyes (6) draw in a false crease line and use pale shadows.

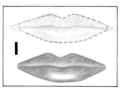

1

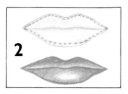

2

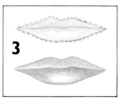

3

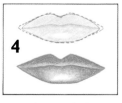

4

It is easy to give your mouth a new shape with clever application of lipstick. Cover the lips with a thin trace of foundation or powder before penciling in a new lip line. The drawings show how to correct a wide (1), full (2), thin (3) and drooping (4) mouth.

To tidy an eyebrow, first brush the hair upward away from the roots. Pluck out any stragglers from underneath and then pencil in the new shape with light strokes.

Tip 50: *Pick the Perfect Foundation*

Foundations are designed to even out skin tone and give the complexion a "flawless" look. A common mistake is to use foundation to give the skin color, which leads to an unsightly "tide mark" between the face and neck. Modern day foundations are cleverly designed not to clog the pores by allowing skin to "breathe." Some are even self-adjusting and adapt to your own natural tone. However, choosing the right foundation for your complexion can be a battle.

Color

Always seek the advice of counter staff when choosing a foundation. Skin comes in different tone – blues, pinks, olives and blacks with many variations in between. While testing for the right color on the inner wrist is a good indicator of whether a shade is flattering for you, it isn't foolproof. Sales staff will test a variety of shades on your cheeks, blending carefully until the true shade matches your own tones.

As a general rule, pink tones are best for sallow skins. A beige-toned foundation is preferable for a pink complexion. If you are blessed with – or think you suffer from – a really highly colored, florid complexion, this can be toned down with an "undercoat" of green-tinted moisturizer applied evenly before you put on your foundation and powder.

Olive and dark skins rarely need more than perhaps a hint of a copper-toned foundation in winter. Very dark skin luckily needs nothing more than plenty of moisturizer to correct any tendency to flaking and dryness. It is worth experimenting with different shades to see which one suits you best.

Texture

Foundations come in various textures: lightweight, medium and heavy coverage. As a general rule, if your skin is young or blemish-free, light coverage will be more flattering, a medium weight is good for winter months when skin needs more coverage, and heavy weight is really only for those with very poor complexions.

While foundations have come a long way since pancake and powder days, it can still be awkward finding your exact match. It will pay off to have help from a counter consultant, but if you are left to your own devices, follow these simple rules to get it right the first time.

• Take three shades that you think might be right for your skin color – one a shade up, one a shade down and one you think is your own tone – and blend each one on your jawbone. The one that is the right shade is the one you can't see!

• Remember that foundation is not to give the skin color – blush does that job. Foundation is used to even out the skin tone so your face looks flawless and smooth.

• "Tide marks" are the demarcation lines between face and neck caused by incorrectly colored foundation or a foundation that has been insufficiently blended.

• If choosing an off-the-shelf foundation, try the newer "color adapting" ones that will regulate to your tone.

• Look for custom blend counters at department stores that will match your exact color and make up a foundation for you there and then.

• Test and apply your shades in natural daylight; department store lighting does nothing for your tone, and to get a true reflection of how perfect the match is, stand outside with a mirror.

Use your fingertips to apply liquid foundation evenly over your face, then blend so that there is no visible line between made-up and unmade-up areas.

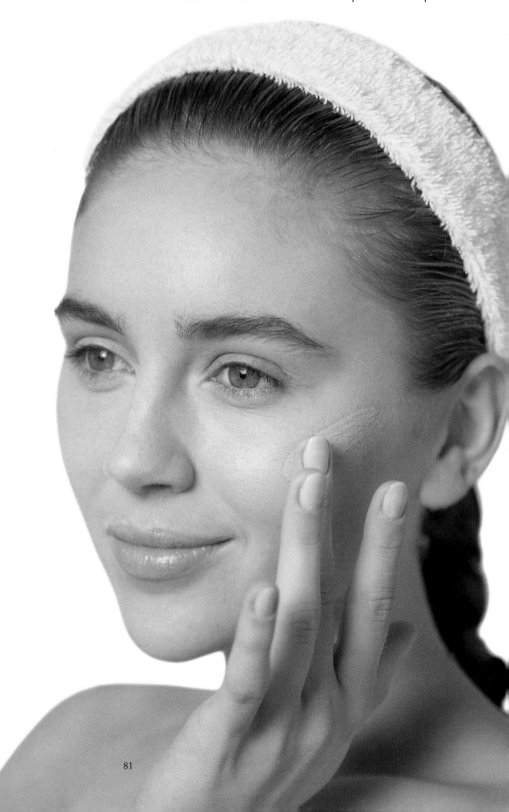

Tip 51: *Mascara and Eyeliner*

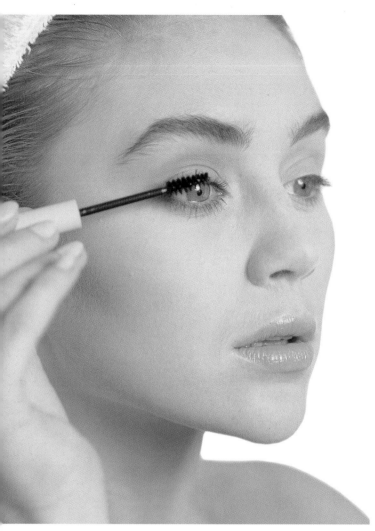

Mascara is applied for longer-looking, darker and more luxuriant lashes. A wand applicator is easiest to use. Apply several coats, waiting in between for each one to dry.

Mascara

There is no doubt that a layer of mascara on the lashes opens up the eyes, making them seem bigger and more wide awake. Common errors with mascara include over-applying, which leads to clumping and makes the lashes look sticky and clogged, and also using the wrong shade. Deep black mascara on blondes and redheads looks completely unnatural.

Choose Your Product

Waterproof mascaras are difficult to get off the eyes – swiping away at the delicate eye area can harm the skin. Waterproofs are best for sporting activities, on the beach or a long evening, as they tend to smudge less. Mascaras that aren't waterproofed are more easily removed, but can leave a "panda eye" look by smudging the undereye area. Lifting, building and curling mascaras do exactly what their names suggest, so anyone with short lashes can get a longer lash appearance by using these specialized products, rather than adding coat after coat.

Choose Your Color

While black is the most popular shade of mascara, more universally flattering is a medium to dark brown. Black is an intense and dramatic shade, which is fabulous for an evening or party look, but browns look more natural for daywear.

How to Apply

In front of a mirror, take your mascara wand and place it under your upper lashes. Blink down onto the wand. Then, placing the wand above the upper lashes, raise the lashes up to the wand. This coats both sides of the lashes effectively. For lower lashes, gently stroke the wand in a downward direction once or twice.

Eyeliner

Eyeliners are a great way to add color or intensity
to the eyes.

Choose Your Liner

Eyeliners should have a butter-soft consistency – hard liners
drag at the skin and are hard to blend. Khols are suitable
for use on the inner rim of the eyelids and give a dramatic
look. Anyone with small eyes should avoid using liner on
the inner rims as it makes the eyes look even smaller.
Liquid eyeliners are very intense and can be difficult to
apply without wobbling. Look out for white eyeliners that
can be used on the inner rim of the eyes for an instantly
wide-awake and brightening effect.

Application

To apply your liner, ensure that you have a mirror and a
table nearby. Balancing your elbow on the table makes
your hand more stable. By gently opening your lower
eyelid with your free hand, stroke the pencil gently across
the inner rim. For liners on the outer rim, use the same
technique, but instead of opening the rim, close the eye
and softly draw from the inner to the outer lid. Some
eyeliners come with a soft, rubber blender attached
and these are perfect for the less confident as any
imperfections can be blended away. Liquid liners require
a very steady hand. Practice first with soft pencil liners.

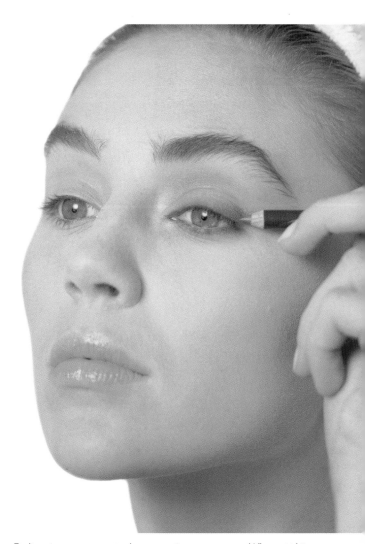

*Eyeliner is a great way to draw attention to your eyes. When applying,
it is essential to keep your hand steady, so balance your elbow
on a table or other firm surface.*

Tip 52: *Eye Shadow*

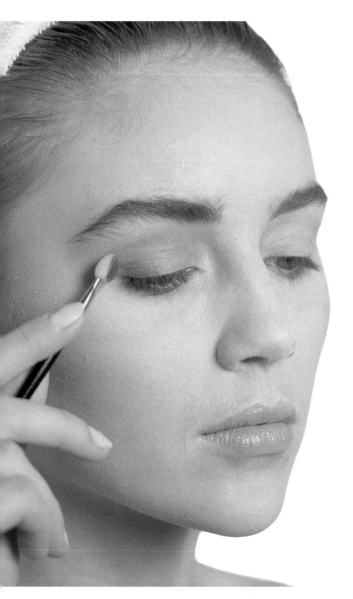

A cotton swab or sponge-tipped applicator will help you apply eyeshadow precisely and evenly over the eye lid area.

Eye coloring is one area where you can afford to experiment without the risk of bankruptcy. The choice is yours – subtle shades of brown and gray or startling but complementary colors.

Eye shadows come in various formats: powder, loose powder, cream and cream-to-powder. Loose powders are the most difficult to use because of their tendency to drop particles, however, the others are much more user-friendly. Powder is probably the simplest of all and is best for oily skin types where the eyelids tend to get greasy. To apply, use a square-tipped brush to pick up color from the palette and then blend onto the lid of the eye. Well-blended shades look more sophisticated because the blending action smoothes out the pigments, giving an even look. Cream eye shadows can give a creased effect, where pools of shadow seep into the natural lines on the lid of the eye. To combat this, use an eye primer first. The advantage of cream shadows is that they can be carefully finger applied, and have a natural blending capacity. Cream-to-powders are the best of both worlds! They go onto the lid with the ease of a cream, but dry to the consistency of a powder. Choose these if you have oil-prone skin. If your skin color is dark, look for deeply pigmented shades that will blend easily and complement your eyes. Lighter colors look un-natural and often have a chalky effect on black skin, but earth tone deep shimmers are a glamorous evening look. For lighter skin, concentrate on a light base shadow, and over the top blend your favorite shades.

Tip 53: *Blush*

Once you have experimented with blush you will realize that it plays an essential part in the art of makeup. It flatters with color and with shape, too, and careful use of it can make the most of your looks.

Blush comes in various formats: powder, cream and tints. It is important to get the correct tone of blush for your skin color and avoid putting on too much color, no matter how washed out you think you look! The natural place for blush is on the apples of the cheeks, where usual flushing would take place; and to find this point, a big smile will naturally push your cheeks out. Powder blush has a tendency to disappear during the day as the particles are brushed off your face; cream blush lasts longer (unless your skin is oily) and has a more blendable and versatile consistency. Tints are translucent pops of color that give a hint of a flush, and are ideal for those who love a minimal or natural look. Black skin should opt for deep rose pinks that give a hint of color to the cheeks, and tints are perfect for this as they don't block out your natural color, but merely glaze over the top. Lighter skin types should stick to earthy tones or neutral pinks.

However much blush you think you need, halve the amount! A common mistake is to apply too much blush, and in the case of powder blush it's almost impossible to reduce the color. Cream blush has the advantage of blending easily, so if you have overdone it dab with a tissue and reblend.

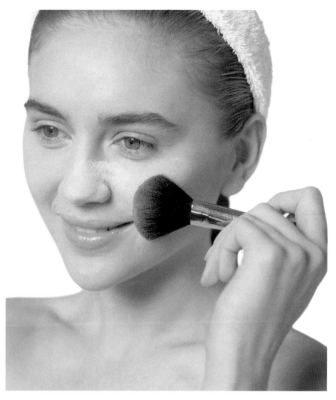

Before applying powder blusher, use a fat brush to dust on powder so that it covers the face, then brush in a downward direction to apply smoothly.

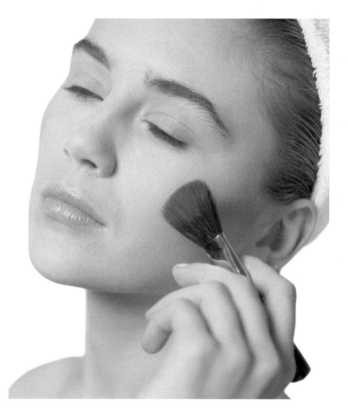

Apply powder blusher over face powder, sweeping color lightly under the cheekbones upward toward the top of the ears.

Tip 54: *Highlighting*

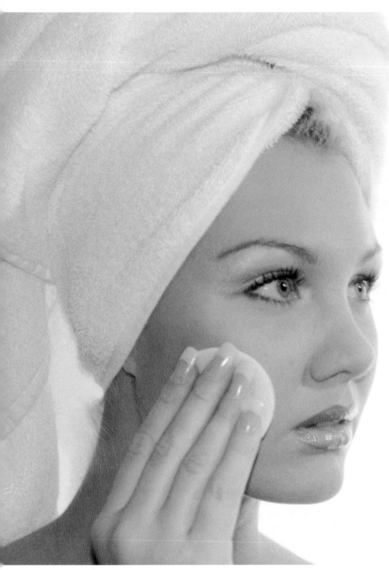

Cream highlighters are perfect for adding definition to your cheekbones. It can be applied with a sponge or your fingers.

Highlighters can be used to brighten, lighten and enhance your face and makeup, as well as placing emphasis on your best features. Two main formulas are available: highlighter pencils and cream highlighter. The advantage of a pencil highlighter is that it is completely controllable. The pencil you buy should have a butter-soft consistency for easy application. Cream highlighter pens work by depositing the cream through a brush at the tip. They're very straightforward to use and have a wide range of applications. They can be used to cover blemishes and uneven color, and many of them contain reflective particles to add a glow. Using a highlighter pencil just below the eyebrow, following the natural brow line, will define your brows and brighten the eye area. Pencils can also be used to shade the middle section of your lower eyelid to give a dazzling, intense appearance to your makeup. Cream highlighters look wonderful

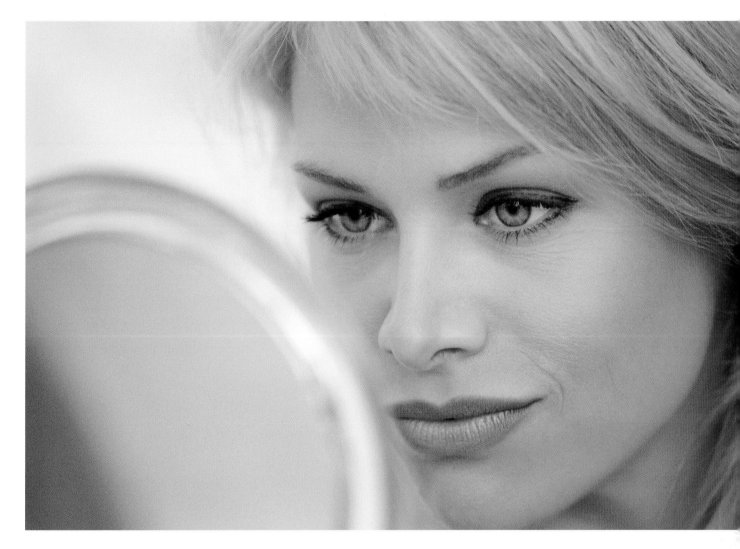

Highlighters can be used to mask blemishes and will give the skin an even, healthy look.

on cheekbones, giving luminosity and emphasizing their qualities, and can be applied with a sponge or your fingers. Dab three tiny dots above the apples of your cheeks and blend to emphasize your cheekbones. The consistency of highlighters vary; some contain a lot of glitter and are only suitable for an evening look, as you can actually see the individual specks of glitter. Shimmer highlighters are also sparkly, but the particles are much finer, giving a more sheer appearance. Try using these on the tips of your shoulders too for more glamour. A highlighting sheen is the safest option of all. Minute particles give a light-catching luster that diffuses fine lines and gives a muted emphasizing effect. Cream highlighters can also be used to lower a high color or to pearlize matte makeup. All skin tones can use highlighters. Dark skin tones suit highlighters with bronze undertones, Asian tones look best with yellow undertones, and very light skin tones are enhanced by white or pinky undertones.

Tip 55: *Lipstick and Gloss*

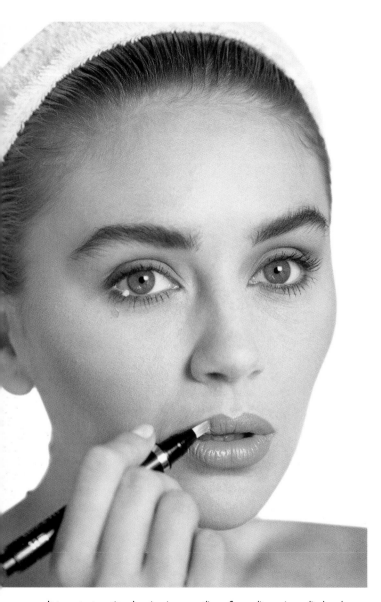

It pays to practice drawing in an outline of your lips using a lip brush. Steady your hand by resting your two lower fingers on your chin if necessary. Recharge the brush and fill in the rest of your lip area; blot and repeat, finishing with gloss.

Your lips at their best are expressive and sensual. Lipstick should enhance these qualities, making them moist, supple, glossy and rosy – never cracked and dry. You can easily improve the shape of your lips by drawing a new outline with a lip pencil or brush. Your choice of lip color can determine the balance of your face. A lighter, more natural shade of lipstick will allow the attention to be focused on the eyes, but if you want to try a different effect, go for a darker lipstick and minimal eye makeup.

The difference between lipstick and lip gloss lies in the density of color and the consistency. Glosses tend to be translucent shades that give a high shine to the lips; whereas lipstick has a full pigmentation and color depth, and has a creamy or matte texture. Glosses are sticky to the touch and often need regular reapplication, whereas lipsticks do not feel tacky and are longer lasting. Lip gloss, clear or delicately tinted, can be used over lipstick to give an added sheen. Alternatively, it can be used by itself to give a dewy, natural look. Many women find that special "long-last" or matte look lipsticks dry out the lips; applying a lip balm under your lipstick can counteract this problem. However, this does hinder adhesion, so don't expect it to last as long.

When buying lipstick, it is best to choose good quality kinds, which will not vanish within five minutes. Although these can be expensive, they are undoubtedly worth the cost. Matching lip pencils are available from most good manufacturers, and they give a lovely, subtle shape to the mouth. Choose a lip color that complements the natural tone of your lips and skin. Black skin tones tend to suit richer shades, such as plums, wines and deep reds, while olive or Asian tones suit light browns, raisins, brown-reds and caramels. White or pink skin tones are enhanced by neutrals, pinks or light browns. Most lip glosses come with their own applicator wand, but if your favorite shade doesn't, invest in a lip brush for even application. Lipsticks are best applied with a brush, even though their shape invites direct application. By putting your lipstick directly onto your lips and pressing both lips together, it is easy to miss outlining the "cupid's bow" at the top of your upper lip. This is such a defining part of the mouth that it should be shown off! Swipe a lip brush over your lipstick several times to get a good amount onto the brush. Then literally fill in your lips with color, ensuring an even application. Gloss needs less precision due to its more "gloopy" consistency, but care should be taken to ensure it doesn't go outside the natural lip line. Look for lipsticks or glosses with SPF (sun protection factor) to protect your lips from burning in hot weather. A favorite makeup artist tip to keep lipstick longer lasting is to apply a first coat, then blot with tissue by placing the tissue between your lips and pressing down, and then applying another coat. You can use a clear gloss over your favorite lipstick to give it more intensity and shine, or mix a little lipstick, using a lip brush, with clear gloss to get a translucent formulation of your shade. Keep lipstick in a cool place as it is prone to melt due to its high oil content.

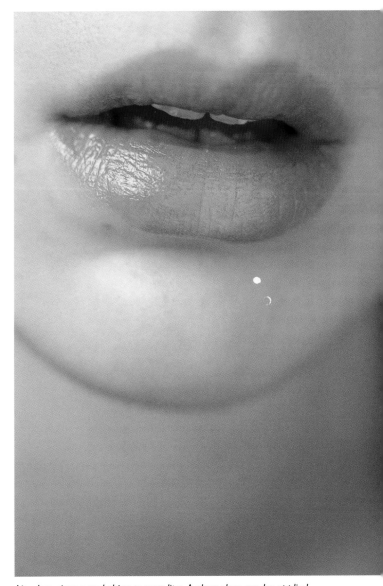

Lip gloss gives a real shine to your lips. A clear gloss can be applied over your favorite lipstick to give it more intensity and shine. Alternatively, you can use a lip brush to mix a little lipstick with clear gloss to get a translucent formulation of your shade.

Tip 56: *Blending Color*

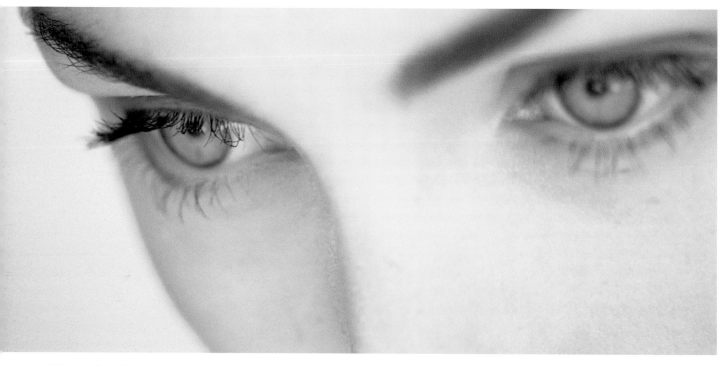

When applying foundation, dab dots of it around your face and gently wipe all over your skin, including your eyelids, with a latex sponge.

When beauty professionals talk about blending color, they mean applying makeup in such a way that it appears seamless with no obvious stops and starts in color. Professional makeup artists can blend cosmetics in such a way that they can literally change your facial shape with visual effects. However, this is makeup at an advanced level. Blending your foundation so it appears completely smooth and natural, and blending your eyes to look seamless is not hard, but the results will be noticeable.

To achieve the best results when blending foundation, you need to use a latex sponge. Apply your foundation in small dots around your face to avoid a block of cover in one place and, using the sponge, wipe gently all over the facial skin, including over the eyelids, ensuring that you take particular care around the eyes. The trick is to keep blending, even if your skin looks perfectly covered. The more you blend the more even and sheer your skin will look. Cream blush blends more easily into skin that has a base of foundation, and this can be done quite easily with your fingertips. Use small amounts and increase if necessary. Eye shadow blending has to be done with an eye shadow brush in order to achieve a precise result. Natural oil on your fingers can actually end up removing your eye shadow rather than blending it, which is why the use of a brush is so crucial. The best way to blend eye makeup is to apply a darker shadow over the top of a lighter one. You may want to fill in the entire eye area with a light shade or highlighter, and then add effect and drama by using a darker color over the top lid. Gentle brushing with your eye shadow brush, particularly in the socket area, will achieve that seamless graduation of color. If it isn't blended enough, just keep going until it is!

Tip 57: *When Less Is More*

Most beauty professionals would say that less is always more! Remember that trends in makeup have moved away from the blues and oranges of the 1980s to more muted, natural looking makeup. Party looks are fun and adventurous, and evening looks allows for color experimentation and all out glamour. However, the harsh light of day is a different story altogether. That hot red that looked so vampy and sophisticated at a party will look way too bright and draining for normal daylight. So, tone it down and remember that the style of makeup you choose should be suited to the occasion. Party makeup will differ from the makeup you choose to wear to the office.

Changing from a full coverage foundation to a tinted moisturizer is a good way to lighten up, as is using a blush tint, and opting for a clear or neutral gloss rather than full color lipstick. By switching your usual black mascara to a brown one, you will still get all the length you need, but just less intensity in color. If you are confident about your skin, then skipping foundation is fine, but keep to a hint of blush if you are pale and be sure to apply sunscreen. You can dab the merest hint of blush on the bridge of your nose to even out your cheek color. Also look out for clear, colorless mascaras that give the lashes a dewy, defined appearance.

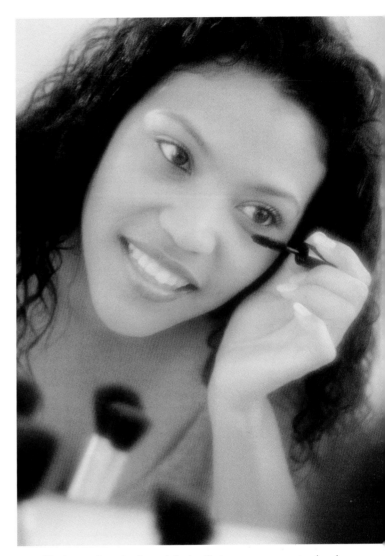

The best makeup is often subtle. It will give you a more natural and sophisticated look.

Tip 58: *Changing the Shape of Your Lips*

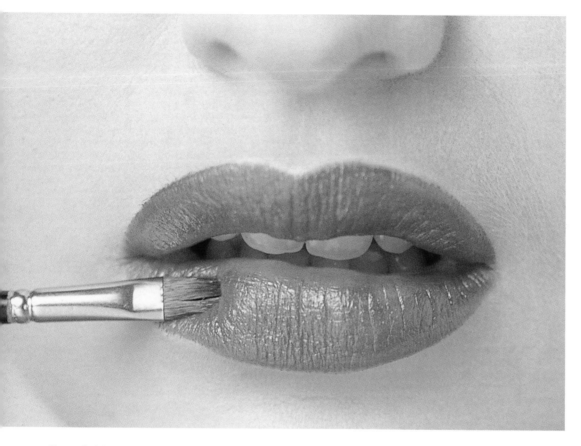

Using a few simple tricks of the trade, lips can be made to look fuller and more sensuous.

Since fashion dictates that full and sensuous lips are the most desirable, using a few tricks of the trade to change your lip shape can help fill out and perfect your pout. To give thin lips a fuller appearance, try using a soft, but thin brown lip pencil to draw gently above the natural lip line following the contours of your mouth. Follow this with a lip pencil the same color as your lipstick to draw over the natural lip line. By gently blending with your finger you can bring these lines together. Pat some loose powder over the top and then fill with lipstick. Remember, this only works by being subtle, so don't make the lines too far apart. A good technique for anyone with full lips is to stick to neutral colors and focus more on using color on your eyes. That way the emphasis on your lips is detracted. If you feel your lips are uneven, try using concealer on a fine brush to bring them more into balance by concealing unevenness. Outline with a natural lip liner, and pat with translucent powder to seal the concealer. Apply your lipstick as normal.

If, on the other hand, you want to minimize your full lips, outline just within the edge of your lips with a lip pencil. Start at the center of the upper lip and stroke down toward each corner. Now do the same for the lower lip. Put some color that is a shade lighter than the pencil onto the lip brush and fill in your lips, starting at the center and working out toward the corners.

Tip 59: *Eyebrow Grooming*

Only pluck hairs below the brow bone and from the bridge of your nose, as regular plucking may eventually stop the follicles from producing hair.

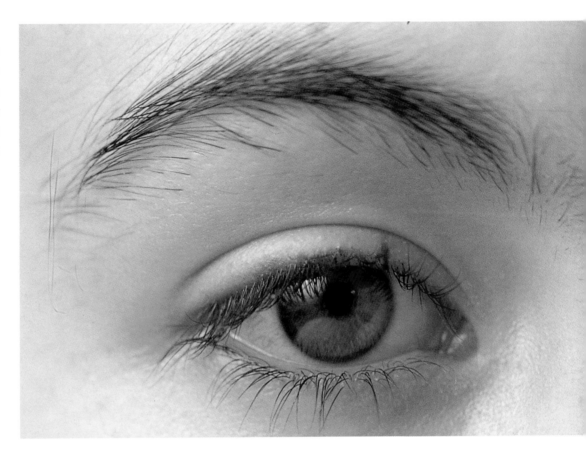

There has never been a stronger style trend than immaculately groomed eyebrows. For those lucky enough to have perfectly arched brows, a slick of petroleum jelly is enough to give them sleekness and stop any stray hairs from sticking up. However, the majority of women have tried at some point to alter their natural brow, with varying degrees of success. A common problem is overplucking — eventually the follicles know when they are beaten and give up producing any hair at all. So, a key point to remember when grooming your brows is not to aim for a thin, unnatural line, but to remove only the hairs from below the brow bone, or any that form between the brows over the bridge of the nose. Long brow hairs can be trimmed with scissors rather than pulled out and smoothed down with a brow wax. Experts recommend plucking your brows after a warm shower as this is when pores are open and the hair removal will be less painful. If you are in any doubt about plucking your own brows, have it done once professionally and then follow their good work during maintenance. Brow pencils give color and depth to lighter brows, but always choose a shade close to your natural hair color.

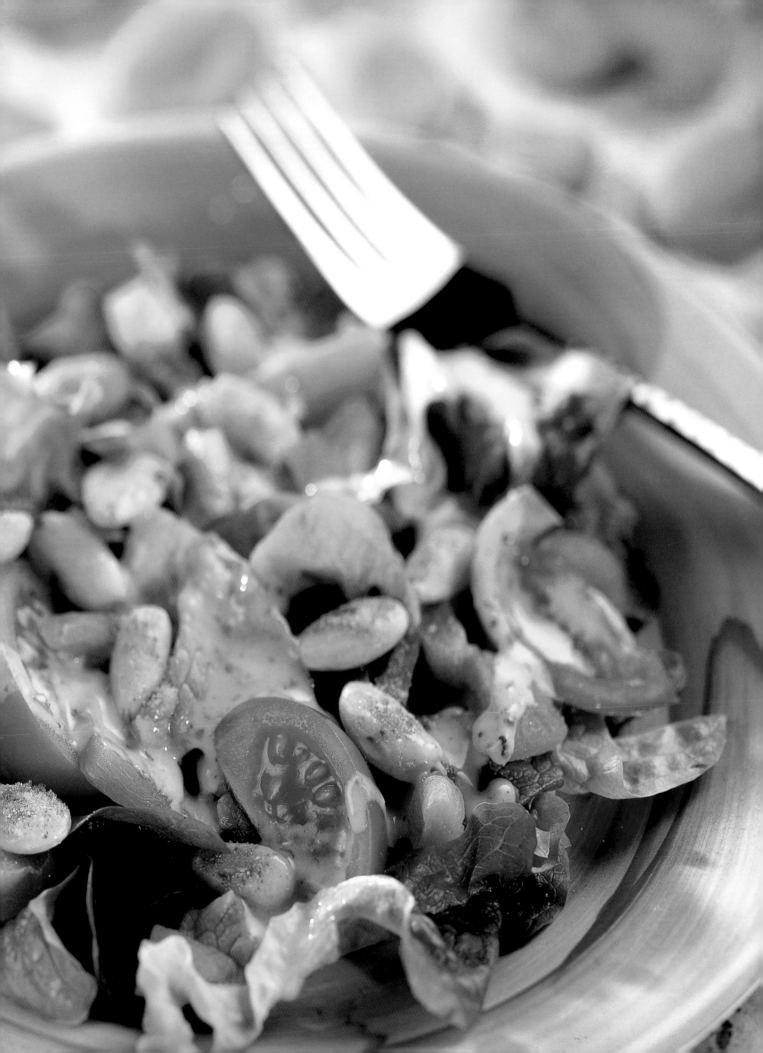

chapter four
HEALTHY
EATING

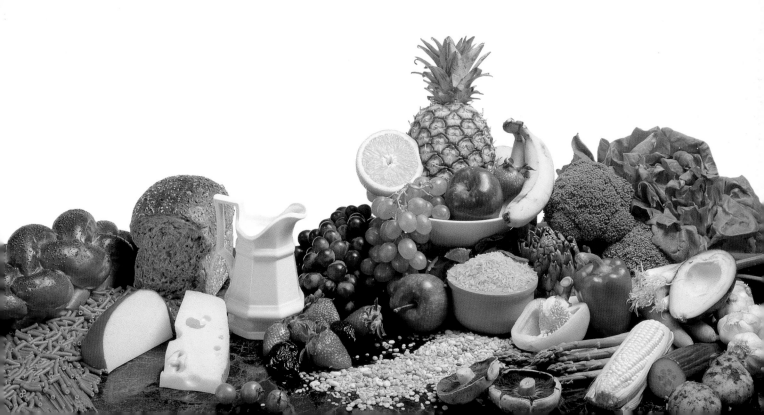

Tip 60: *A Balanced Diet*

Over the last few decades more and more diseases have been linked to our dietary habits and the specific foods that we eat. We now know that, among other risk factors, poor diet is associated with heart disease, some cancers, obesity, hypertension, osteoporosis and anemia to name but a few diseases and ailments.

Surveys also show us that increasing numbers of meals as well as snacks are eaten away from the home, that we tend to graze throughout the day and that families rarely sit down to enjoy a meal together.

People also talk about the stresses of modern day living, coping with ever-busier schedules and feeling unfit and unhealthy. Not surprisingly, all these things are linked, and our feeling of well-being, as well as our physical appearance, is greatly influenced by what we eat. Frequent snacking on high-sugar and high-fat foods gives unhealthy peaks in blood sugar levels, leaves us short of essential vitamins and minerals, and spoils the appetite for more nutritious foods.

While we are probably all well aware of foods to steer clear of, it can be confusing to work out what we should be eating. In a world of celebrity diets and fashionable food fads, uncovering what our bodies really need to stay healthy is a minefield. Food consists of nutrients that include carbohydrates, proteins and fats, as well as vitamins and minerals. Avoiding certain foods will protect your body – in particular your heart – from disease and becoming overweight. As obesity levels continue to soar, however, it is clear that the message of how to adequately enrich your body without barraging it with high levels of unsaturated fats and salt, has stayed a mystery to some. Without a doubt, there is a connection between eating well and looking good. A woman with a well balanced diet has glowing skin, shiny hair and plenty of energy. If you don't have these attributes, look carefully at what you eat. However, this has to be balanced with a realistic expectation; although most of us are aware that organic foods (those produced without the use of pesticides) are likely to be better for our health, it isn't always possible or affordable to stick to. Dietary experts will always say that to deny yourself certain food groups will only contribute to making any eating plan difficult. It is okay to indulge in chocolate or cookies every now and again, but if they make up a large proportion of what you eat in a day, your body is likely to show it in terms of high weight level and poor skin. Another reason that food can become our enemy instead of our friend is portion size. Your plate should never be overflowing or piled high. Once you have begun to eat oversize amounts, your expectation of how much food you actually need to function effectively becomes distorted. Bodies that are carrying excess weight just don't function properly. The joints are under considerable strain to bear excess weight, as well as the heart, which needs to work harder to keep blood flowing around your body.

A diet consisting of all the major food groups is a healthy one. Remember to keep your consumption of high sugar and high fat foods to a minimum.

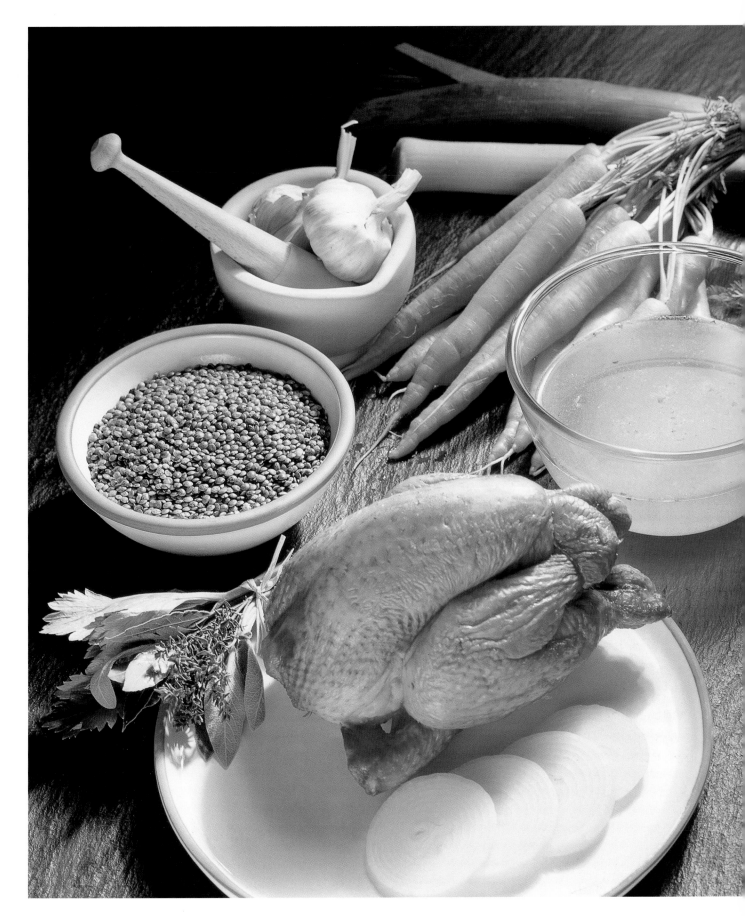

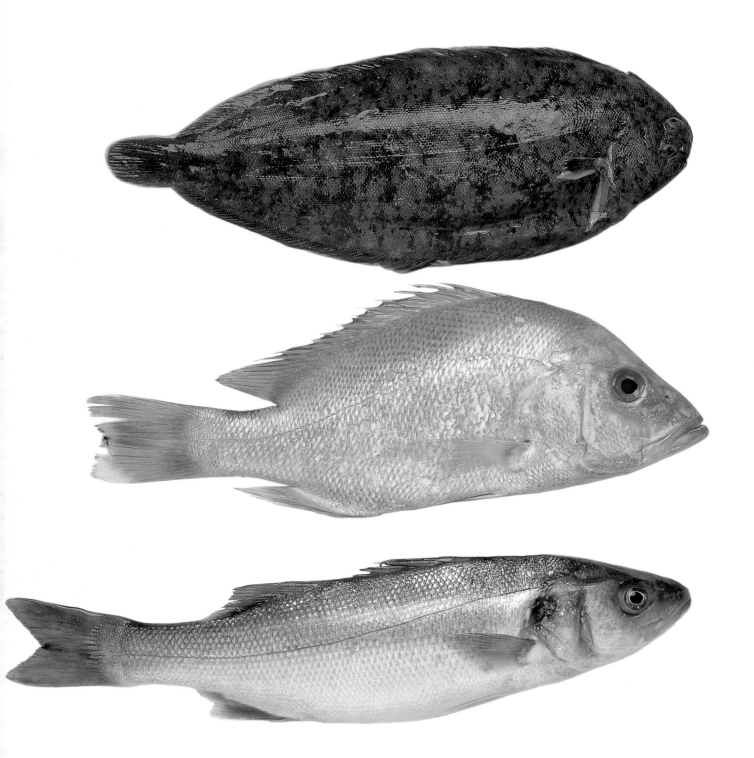

Fish should be a part of your balanced diet. It is the best source of
compounds known as omega-3 fatty acids, which help reduce the
stickiness of blood, and the consumption of two or three servings of fish
a week is related to a lower risk of heart attack. Omega-3 fatty acids
are particularly prevalent in oily fish.

One of many excuses for not eating a healthy, balanced diet is lack of time, and with the ready availability of convenience foods, nutrition loses out in the time versus health dilemma. Planning ahead is the key to eating healthy foods – if there is nothing in the refrigerator it's all too easy to get take out. Have a good stock of basic, healthy foods, such as fresh vegetables and herbs, pasta, fruit and cheese, and throwing together a quick supper can take less time than waiting for your take out to be delivered.

The USDA's new MyPyramid symbolizes a personalized approach to healthy eating and physical activity. It is a tool to help you make healthier food and physical activity choices for a healthy lifestyle that is consistent with dietary guidelines. Each person has a Pyramid that is right for them based on their age, sex and physical activity level. For example, for a 2,000-calorie diet, you need 6 ounces of grains, 2½ cups of vegetables, 2 cups of fruit, 3 cups of milk and 5½ ounces (156 g) of meat and beans every day. To find out what you need to eat each day according to your physical activity level go to MyPyramid.gov.

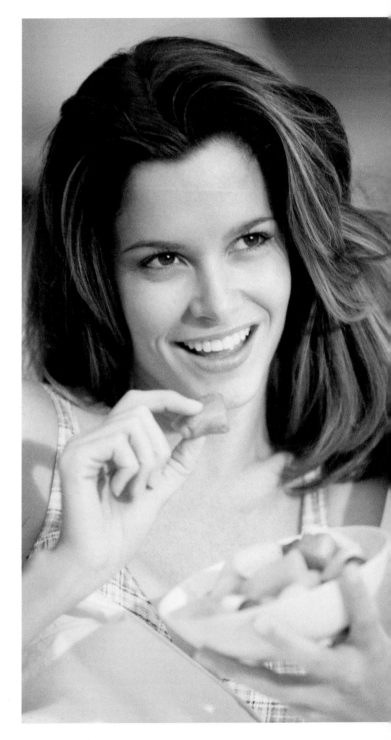

Eating a balanced diet that is high in fruit and vegetables is an essential part of a healthy lifestyle. The USDA's new MyPyramid provides you with personalized information on how much to eat from the different food groups every day.

Tip 61: *Essential Fats, Vitamins & Minerals*

Not all fats are bad; in fact good fats are essential for healthy skin, bones and hair, as well as brain function, the nervous system and hormonal balancing, and are an excellent source of energy. However, the difference between "good" and "bad" fats are whether they fall into the saturated or unsaturated category. Fat is made up of two compounds – fatty acids and glycerol. The fatty acids may be saturated, monounsaturated or polyunsaturated, and different foods contain a mixture of each.

Too much saturated fat is potentially damaging to the body; it increases the risk of heart disease and Type 2 diabetes. Saturated fat raises the levels of undesirable low-density lipoprotein (LDL) cholesterol in the blood, and dietary

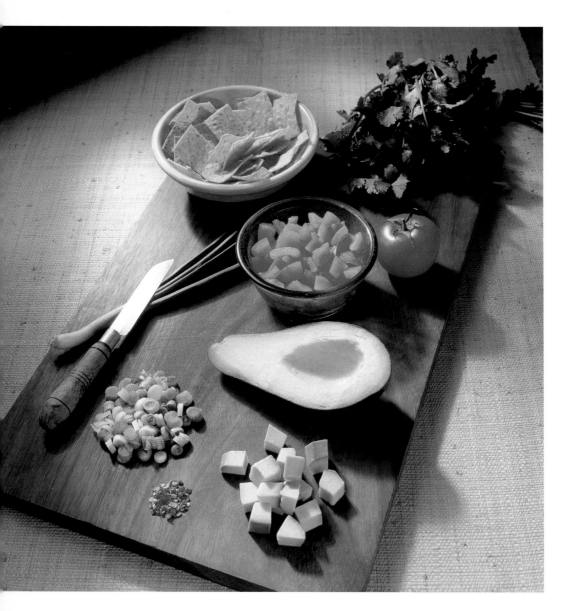

Compared to other vegetables, avocados are high in fat and calories, but they contain mostly monounsaturated fats, which help to protect against heart disease. They are also rich in vitamin E, which is an important antioxidant in the human body.

recommendations are that no more than 10 percent of total calories should be provided by saturated fatty acids. Conversely, monounsaturated fatty acids have a tendency to lower the levels of undesirable cholesterol in the blood and raise the level of more beneficial forms. the net result is that individuals whose diets rely upon monounsaturated fatty acids, rather than saturated fats, are less likely to develop hardening of the arteries (atherosclerosis). Olive and canola oils contain mostly monounsturated fatty acids, although nuts, avocados, meat and dairy products contain some too. Polyunsaturated fats and oils are still preferred to saturated fats but do not have the same benefits as monounsaturated fats. Polyunsaturated fats are found mainly in sunflower and corn oils and in some vegetables. Vegetable oils are often used in the preparation of shortening and margarine. Part of the process is known as hydrogenation, which changes the overall structure of the fat. Substances called trans-fatty acids are produced, and these behave in a similar way to saturated fatty acids. These can be found in many processed and fast foods, and should be avoided as much as possible.

Essential fats cannot be made by the body and should comprise 20 percent of your daily food intake. Essential fatty acids (omega-3 and omega-6) are called essential because our bodies cannot function without them. Find them in abundance in food groups such as oily fish (salmon, trout, mackerel and tuna), and nuts and seeds. Oils such as olive oil, flaxseed oil and walnut oil are good providers of fatty acids.

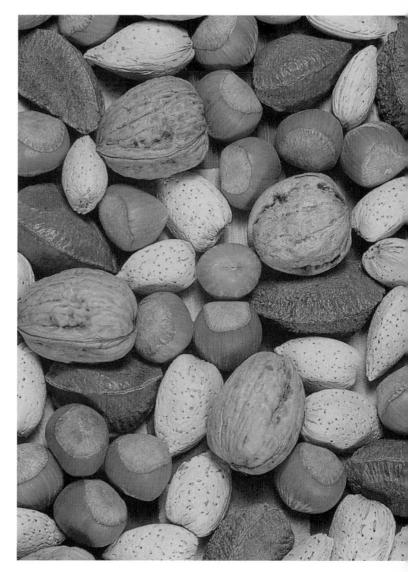

Nuts, along with oily fish and seeds, are a good source of essential fatty acids.
They are also a good source of protein.

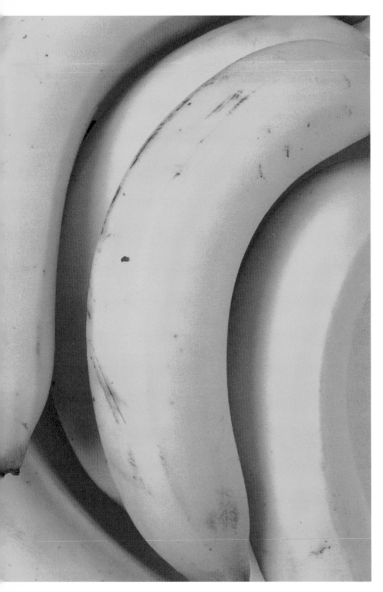

Bananas are a good source of carbohydrates, which will keep you full of energy. They are also high in the mineral potassium. The other major minerals required by your body in significant quantities are calcium, phosphorous, chloride, magnesium, zinc, iron and sodium.

When it comes to maintaining a healthy vitamin supply, if you eat at least five portions of fresh fruit and vegetables a day, you should not be deficient in vitamins, although many people prefer to take a vitamin supplement to make sure. Vitamins A, D, E, B and C are thought to be the essential vitamins. Vitamin A is vital for the body's growth and development, including eyesight and reducing infections. Orange, yellow and dark green fruits and vegetables, as well as liver, all contain high quantities. Vitamin D aids mineral absorption and good bone health, and is found in foods such as eggs, oily fish and cod liver oil, but most vitamin D comes from sunlight. While vitamin E is thought to protect against heart disease and possibly some cancers, its healing function is vital to reduce inflammation in the body. Foods that have a high source of this vitamin include legumes and beans, whole-wheat flour and leafy green vegetables. The group of B vitamins are vital for nervous system health and to help release energy from the food we eat. Luckily they are found in a variety of foods. Included in your vitamin B–rich diet should be oats, cereals and bread, whole-grains, beans and legumes. They are also found in fruit and vegetables, and high sources from this food group include mushrooms, bananas, avocados and watercress. A lack of vitamin C can lead to bleeding gums, poor skin and hair functions and a poor immune system (constant coughs and colds). Strong dietary sources of vitamin C are dark fruits, such as blueberries, blackberries and blackcurrants, peppers and brussel sprouts. Finally, and particularly in pregnancy, folic acid plays a vital role in the development of cells and pregnant women are often advised to take a supplement. Foods that are rich in folic acid include leafy, green vegetables, oranges and cereals.

Tip 62: *Water – Staying Hydrated*

Without realizing it, many of us are dehydrated. Water is one of the cheapest and most abundant beauty aids around, and drinking plenty will show not only in your skin but your energy levels too. Drinking too much tea, alcohol, coffee and colas has a diuretic effect – making you need to pass water more – and so actually have a dehydrating effect on the body, leading to fatigue and constipation. Experts recommend drinking about eight glasses of water per day. Obviously, in hot weather or after exercise this should be increased. Not everyone finds this amount of fluid easy to cope with, but after a while your body will get used to the extra amount of water and regulate itself accordingly. Air conditioned or centrally heated homes and offices also have a dehydrating effect, so be sure to have a good supply on hand. By flushing toxins throughout the body, water acts as an effective system cleanser – not having enough water can lead to headaches, slowing down the metabolic system and cause urine or kidney infections.

Keep bottled or filtered water available at all times, and sip throughout the day. When you wake up, start the day with a glass of water, then drink another glass while you are getting dressed. At about 11 a.m., instead of reaching for the coffee pot, have a little freshly squeezed orange juice topped up with mineral water, and the same around 4 p.m. Pour yourself a glass of water to sip while you are having a soak in the bathtub in the evening, and have another glass before you go to bed. That's six – just one more glass each with your lunch and evening meal and you've hit the target. Not that difficult, is it?

Drinking plenty of water (around six to eight glasses a day) keeps our kidneys functioning correctly and removes toxins from the body.

Tip 63: *Fruits and Vegetables*

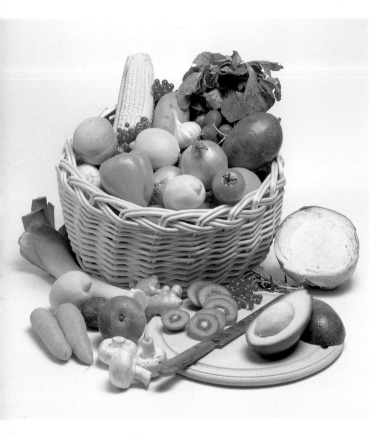

At least five portions of fresh fruit and vegetables a day are recommended. Although fresh is always best, canned, frozen and dried also count. Try to eat as wide a variety of fruit and vegetables as possible.

Fruits and vegetables are a delicious way to stay healthy. They are packed with fiber, vitamins and minerals, and due to their low calorie count need not be rationed in any way. Five portions a day are recommended, although this is the minimum amount; bear in mind that if you don't have fresh produce easily available, canned, frozen or dried counts, too, although it is always best to eat fresh fruit and vegetables when possible.

Most vegetables are naturally low in fat. None of them contain cholesterol. In their natural state they are low-calorie foods. You can serve vegetables in a number of delicious ways including broiled, roasted, baked, steamed, stewed or braised. Just remember to avoid adding too much oil, butter or cheese to the dishes you select. The beauty of fruit, apart from its obvious health benefits, is that it is so convenient and portable – it makes a quick and easy snack. It provides energy in the form of natural sugars and is a nutritious way to keep up blood sugar levels throughout the day.

It is important to remember that fruit and vegetable juices will only count as one portion toward your recommended

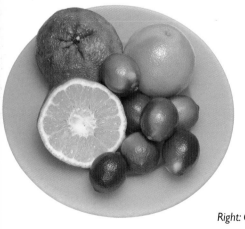

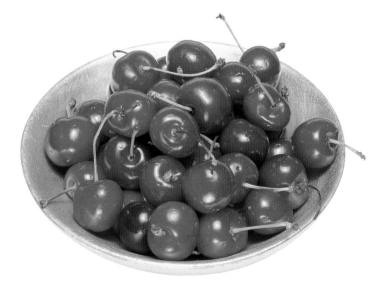

Left: Citrus fruits such as limes and grapefruit are high in vitamin C and can be used to flavor other foods. Right: Cherries are a delicious source of vitamin C.

five a day. Experts suggest that grouping your fruits and vegetables by color ensures that you get a good and varied range. Ensure you choose from greens, reds and a piece of citrus fruit to get a good variety. Fruits and vegetables are the ultimate superfood – one orange can give you up to 93 percent of your needed vitamin C for the day! Both are full of antioxidants, which provide a strong protective role for your body, helping to lower bad fats in the blood and protect heart muscles, arteries and cells. Antioxidants effectively "clean up" the body's toxins and harmful substances. Red grapes, kiwi fruit and berries are also high in the powerful antioxidant vitamin C. Green vegetables are known to be high in iron, essential for healthy blood cells. To get the optimum nutrition from vegetables, experts recommend that steaming is a more vitamin-conserving method of cooking than boiling, as much of the vegetable's vitamin content actually enters the water or is destroyed at a high temperature. Steaming preserves more active vitamins and minerals. The best way to obtain the most from your fruits and vegetables, however, is to eat them raw. Obviously, in the case of some fruits and vegetables – such as potatoes – cooking is the only way to make them palatable! But, where possible, try to eat some portions of raw vegetables. Carrots, celery, cauliflower, tomatoes and cucumber are some of the easier ones to remember, but shelled peas, peppers and onions can all be eaten raw too. Keeping a ready prechopped and prepared amount of vegetables in an airtight box in the fridge means you always have a healthy snack on hand if you become hungry between meals. If you aren't keen on vegetables, try eating them with a low-fat dip to spice them up a bit.

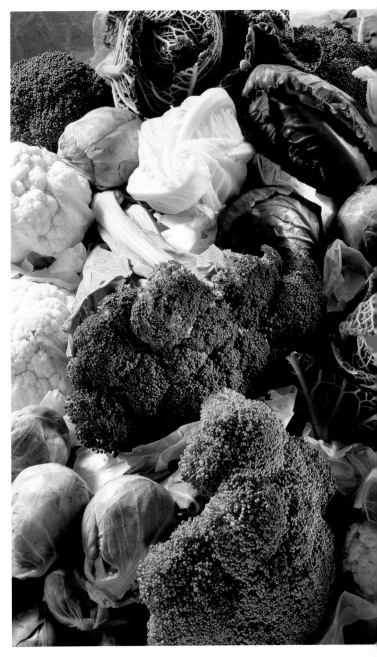

Try steaming your vegetables the next time you serve them. This will ensure that they retain more of their vitamins and minerals.

Tip 64: *Protein and Fiber*

Fiber has an enormous impact on health. It helps to prevent against disease such as bowel cancer, reduces stomach acid and lowers the levels of cholesterol in your blood. Some scientists believe that certain foods contain toxins or chemicals that may induce cancerous changes in the lining of the colon. It is thought that by speeding the passage of food through the intestine, fiber reduces the time during which these chemicals can have this effect. A diet rich in fiber will also promote healthy bowel function. Foods rich in fiber include whole-wheats, brown rice, grains and fruit and vegetables. However, if your body isn't used to lots of fiber, there can be some side effects, including bloating and excess gas. The key is to introduce fiber-rich foods into your diet slowly, allowing your digestive system to get used to dealing with higher levels. You may find that you need to increase your hydration levels by drinking more water as fiber absorbs liquid. The

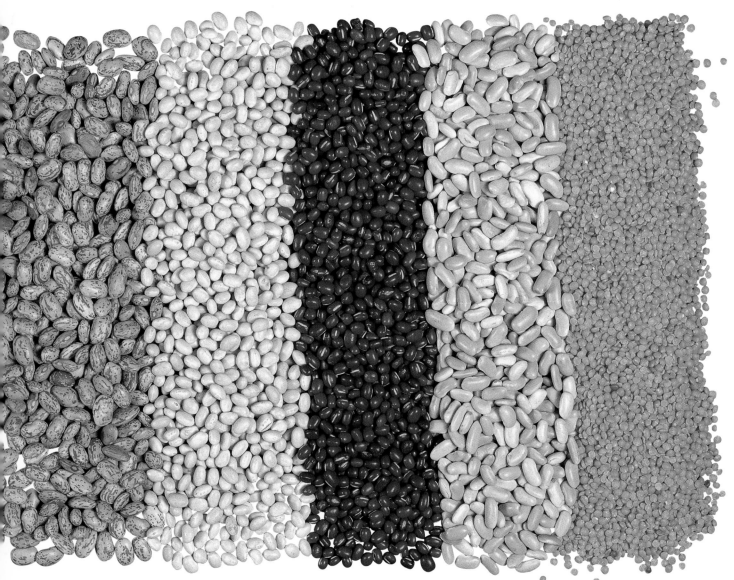

two types of fiber – soluble and insoluble – act in different ways. Soluble fiber, found in foods such as oats, beans and barley, is thought to lower blood cholesterol, while insoluble fiber, found in whole-wheat cereals, rice and many fruits and vegetables, promotes bowel function to ward against bowel cancer.

Protein is an essential daily dietary requirement. Without a certain amount of protein our muscles and bones start to lose their build. Proteins can come in the form of animal or vegetable fat, but a very beneficial protein is soy, which has been found by experts to lower cholesterol. Beans are an excellent source of protein; as is brown rice, lentils and any other legumes. Nuts can also provide good amounts of protein – try to include brazil nuts, peanuts and pine nuts in your diet, but be wary of their high fat content if you are dieting. Meat also provides protein, and rather than always buying regular grocery store steak, consider free-range or organic chicken or turkey, and organic lamb, pork or beef. Tofu, cheese and low-fat milk are also excellent protein sources. Free-range eggs are also a good source, and incredibly versatile to cook with. Consider omelets, scrambled eggs or a good, old-fashioned boiled egg with whole-wheat toast for breakfast. Some studies have suggested that a high intake of protein-rich foods can help people to experience fullness more quickly, which leads to them needing fewer calories during an average day.

Left: Beans and lentils are the seeds from pod-producing plants and are a nutritious meat alternative as they are a good source of protein. They are rich in fiber, including soluble fiber, which helps maintain healthy cholesterol levels.

Above: shellfish such as these mussels are a very good source of protein. However, shellfish, unlike other types of fish, does contain relatively high amounts of cholesterol, so should be eaten only occasionally.

Tip 65: *Carbohydrates*

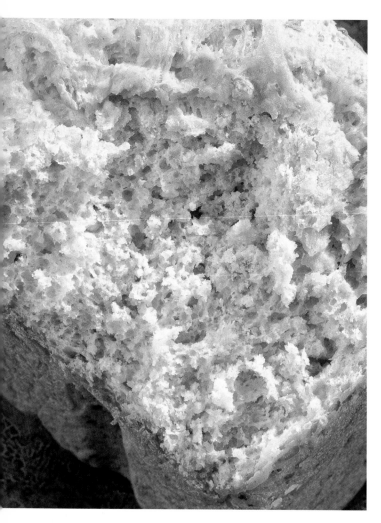

In essence, carbohydrates are sugars and starches in food that provide us with energy and are found predominantly in bread, pasta and sugary foods, such as cookies and cakes. The body has only a limited ability to produce sugar in the bloodstream from substances other than carbohydrates. This means that consuming carbohydrates is essential for energy. While low-carb diets have hit the headlines as sure-fire ways to lose weight, it means the body turns instead to protein to find energy, meaning less is available for essential functions like growth and repairing body tissues. Conversely, too many carbohydrates in the diet can lead to excess weight gain, in which case fiber-rich foods are felt to be more helpful. Carbohydrates should not be perceived as the enemy – there are plenty of nutrient-rich carbohydrate sources, including whole-grain bread, cereal, rice, pasta and also fruit and vegetables.

Choose nutrient-rich carbohydrates such as whole-grain or multi-grain breads, bagels, brown rolls and brown pasta, to accompany your meals. These provide a longer lasting energy without a blood sugar slump.

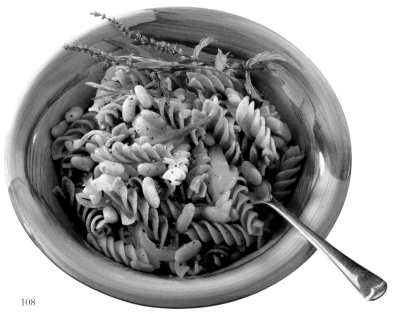

Tip 66: *Dairy Products*

"Dairy products" is one of those confusing categories of foods that, depending upon who you ask, the view upon whether or not it is good for you will vary. Some experts say that dairy is mucus-making, a contributor to skin complaints and high in fats. Others will say that it is an excellent, healthful food source. What can't be denied, however, is the important role of the mineral calcium – contained in abundance in dairy products – in strengthening bones and teeth. Dairy food does not include butter, margarine or cream, which falls into the fat and sugar categories. Foods from the dairy family include cheese, yogurt and milk. Some non-dairy foods, such as dark leafy vegetables, soy milk and sesame seeds are also calcium-rich. Bones continue to benefit from the strengthening effects of calcium well into your 30s, and a lack of calcium can lead to brittle bones in old age. It is particularly important for teenagers and children who are still growing to have enough calcium in their diets. Worries about dairy produce containing a lot of fat can be counteracted by choosing the low-fat options; these contain the same high-calcium content as their fattier counterparts.

Above: Cheese is very high in fat, so should be consumed in moderation. Where possible, use low-fat alternatives.

Below: Milk (center) is an excellent source of calcium. Try to use low-fat skimmed milk rather than whole milk. Heavy creams (left and right) is classed in the fat and sugar category rather than the dairy product category.

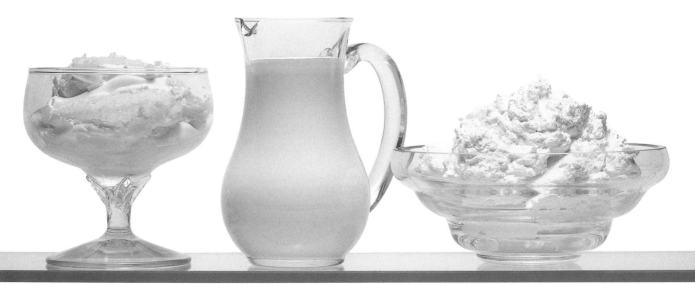

Tip 67: *Sugar and Chocolate*

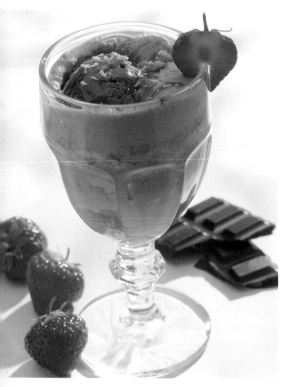

Sugary foods such as ice cream are often high in fat, which can lead to weight gain if consumed too often. A healthier source of sweetness is fruit, which is high in natural sugars.

Sugar is a carbohydrate and a source of energy, but dieticians describe sugar as "empty calories," providing no nutritional value, but lots of calorific value. Sugar comes in various forms: brown, white, raw, corn syrup or even honey. The trouble with sugar, however, is that it is often found in food that contains high amounts of fat such as cookies, cake and ice cream. Sugar also has an impact on other parts of the body, such as teeth, causing decay. Processed foods tend to contain high levels of sugar in order to give taste, bulk and to act as a preservative. Anyone who eats a chocolate bar when they are hungry knows that following the initial feeling of fullness there is an energy dip. Natural sugars, contained in fruit and vegetables give a more sustaining, long lasting energy source. It is easy to eat too much sugar without realizing it, which is why it's important to check the ingredient list on any processed foods. Chocolate, however, while high in sugars, is thought more and more to have many health benefits, so the news for sugar lovers isn't all bad! Of course, chocolate should be eaten in moderation. The nutritional value of chocolate varies according to recipe, and it's thought that dark chocolate is of more nutritional value. But chocolate contains protein, fat, vitamin E, calcium, phosphorous, magnesium, copper, iron and phytochemicals, or plant extracts, mainly from the cocoa bean. This doesn't mean you should indulge in lots of chocolate bars, but what it does mean is that a small amount of dark chocolate included in your regular diet may be beneficial rather than detrimental to your health.

Beware of processed chocolate bars that also contain other ingredients, such as toffee or nuts, as this automatically sends the calorie count skyward. Organic dark chocolate is a sensible and healthy eating choice. There is no evidence to suggest that eating chocolate contributes to acne or breakouts, and despite the obvious benefits of chocolate, it shouldn't be thought of as a "health food," but more a luxury food to be eaten sparingly.

The consumption of high-sugar foods usually spells disaster for energy levels. These foods cause rapid rises in blood sugar that can cause the body to overcompensate, leading to problems with low blood sugar (hypoglycemia) and low levels of physical and mental energy later on.

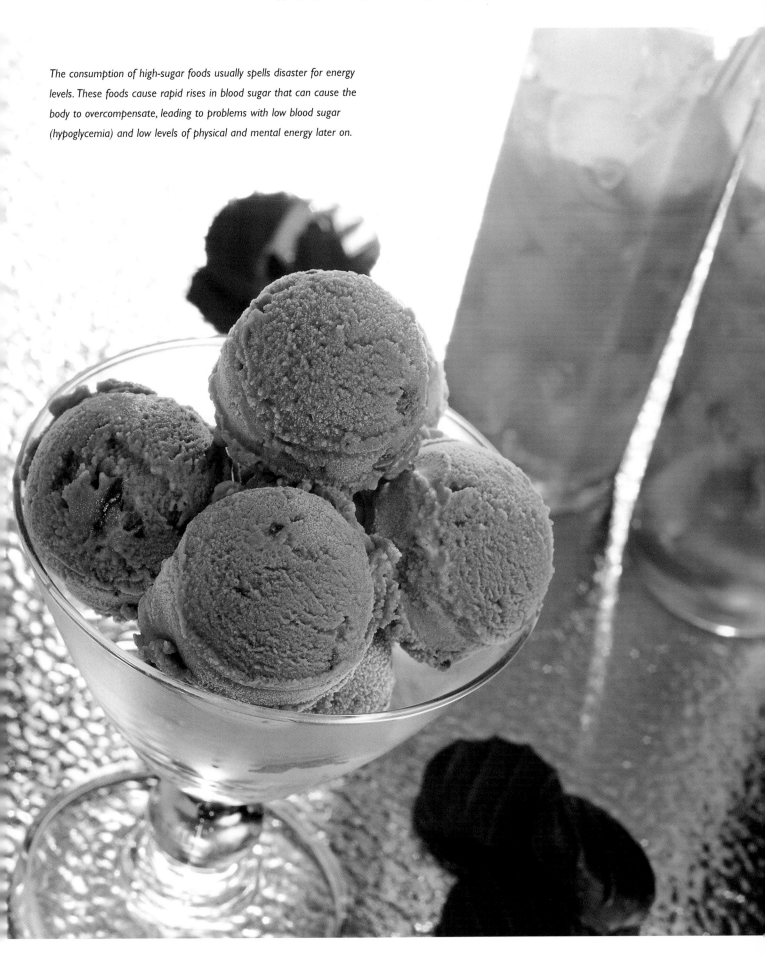

Tip **68:** *Additives and Processed Foods*

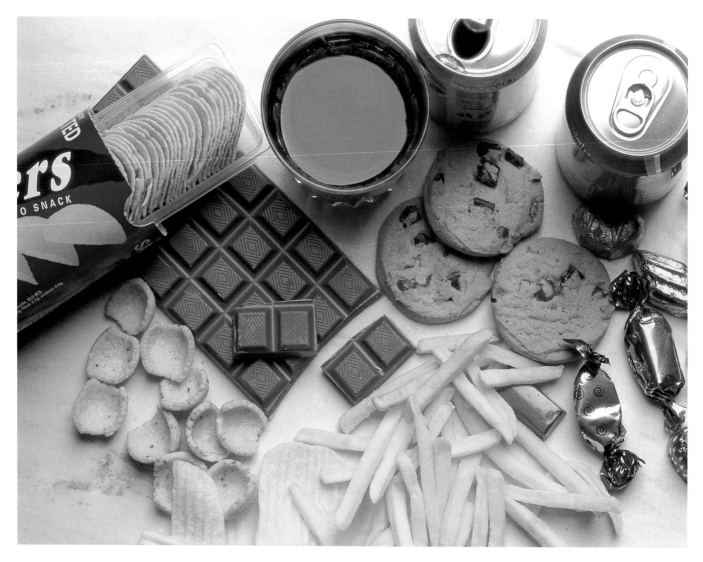

In its broadest sense, a food additive is any substance added to food. Technically, the term refers to "any substance the intended use which results or may reasonably be expected to result – directly or indirectly – in its becoming a component or otherwise affecting the characteristics of any food." This definition includes any substance used in the production, processing, treatment, packaging, transportation or storage of food. On top of this, there are color additives, which are added to food to make it look more visually appealing.

If a substance is added to a food for a specific purpose in that food, it is referred to as a direct additive. For example, the low-calorie sweetener aspartame, which is used in beverages, puddings, yogurt, chewing gum and other foods, is considered a direct additive. Many direct additives are identified on ingredient labels. If an additive has been given approval by a government food standard agency, this is because it is thought to be safe. In the United States, the Food and Drug Administration (FDA) is responsible for approving the safety of additives in food and other products, such as cosmetics. Lists of approved additives do change and new discoveries of potentially harmful additives are on the increase, so although the majority of additives are likely to be perfectly safe, an increasing number of people are choosing to avoid them altogether.

When you read the ingredient listings on a package of processed food, you may find that it contains colors, artificial sweeteners, emulsifiers, stabilizers and preservatives. Added to food to perform specific functions, there are also a number of natural additives, such as beetroot, used as a colorant. Additives are used in processed food to keep it looking or tasting better, to give food a longer shelf life or to enhance the flavors. Additives have been linked in the media to certain illnesses, most commonly cancer, with several major players in the safety question group. These include monosodium glutamate, used in savory processed foods, which is thought to destroy nerve cells and has caused cancers in animal testing. Aspartame is an artificial sweetener 200 times sweeter than sugar, and while manufacturers insist that it is safe, experts think it may cause neurological damage. Saccharine, another popular artificial sweetener, has already been banned in several countries, thought to interfere with digestive function and linking to DNA damage in animal testing. Sulfur dioxide is a common ingredient in soft drinks, and has been found to contribute to gastric problems such as nausea and diarrhea.

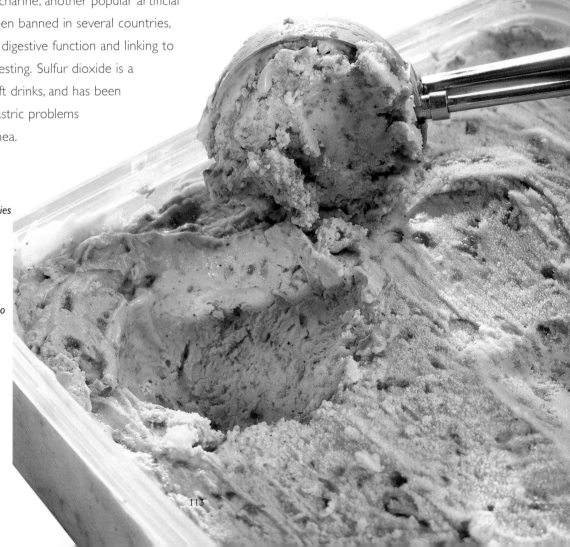

Above left and right: Processed convenience foods such as cookies and candy are high in artificial sweeteners, colors and preservatives, and should be eaten only very occasionally. Indeed, the healthiest thing to do is cut them out of your diet completely.

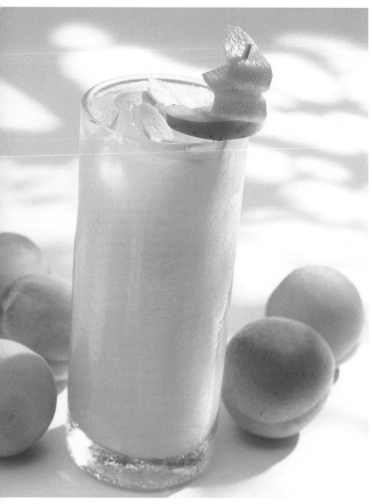

Instead of sugary soft drinks that are high in additives, try drinking fresh squeezed juices, which are not only high in vitamins and minerals, but also in taste.

Artifical colors like D&C Yellow No. 10 and FD&C Yellow No. 6, which can be found in processed foods such as ice cream and soft drinks, are already restricted in some countries. The colorings have been linked to asthma and hyperactivity, as well as some cancers. Recent media attention has uncovered a cancer risk in a chemical food dye called Sudan 1 (also known as Solvent Orange R), commonly found in chilli powder and processed foods. Although researchers have discovered that the presence of Sudan 1 in foods can contribute to an increased risk of cancer, if you have eaten foods containing Sudan 1, there is no need for alarm. The risk found is very small, but the chemical has been removed from food agency "safe lists" and should no longer appear in any food sold.

All these food additives are found in processed foods, meaning that in order to avoid any potential harm from chemicals, it is important to make your food choices carefully. Where possible, avoid prepackaged meals and junk food – all heavy users of additives. Stick to health-food-store sweets that are labeled additive-free, or that use natural food colorings.

To be completely sure you are getting additive-free food, you will need to look down the organic route. To be certified organic, foods have to be grown in pesticide-free soil and not treated with any chemicals in order to make them look or taste better. Organic foods generally have a rougher or less even appearance, rather than the uniform rows of bright green or red apples or overly-orange carrots that you might find on your supermarket shelf. This, of course, does not affect the quality, although without the use of chemicals, you may find fruits and vegetables slightly smaller and less intense in color. It is safe to say that the further you steer clear of junk foods the further you keep from overprocessed and additive-laden food. Applying common sense in food choices is easy – rely on your instincts. If a food looks too bright, or is an unnatural color, such as blue (there are no truly blue foods; even blueberries are purple in shade), it is highly likely that it contains artificial colorings. Food that contains a high level of chemical additives – particularly sweets, sugary drinks and candies – can also give off an unnatural smell. But your main guidance is labeling. Initially time-consuming to check, you will find that learning what is additive-free becomes quick and natural, allowing you to make better, more healthy food choices.

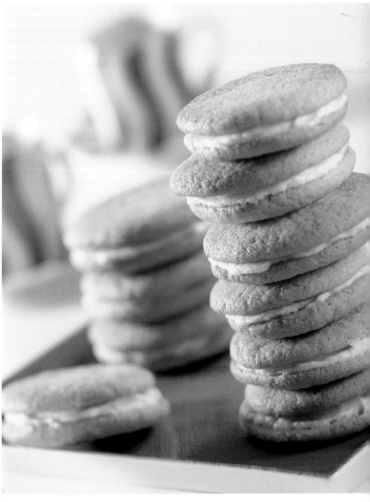

Foods such as cookies are sometimes high in additives. Get into the habit of checking labels before you buy.

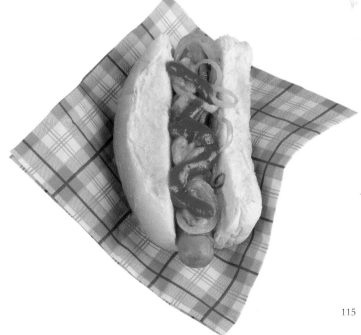

Fast foods such as hot dogs usually contain high levels of additives. As such, they should be cut out of your diet as much as possible.

Tip **69**: *Coffee, Tea & Soft Drinks*

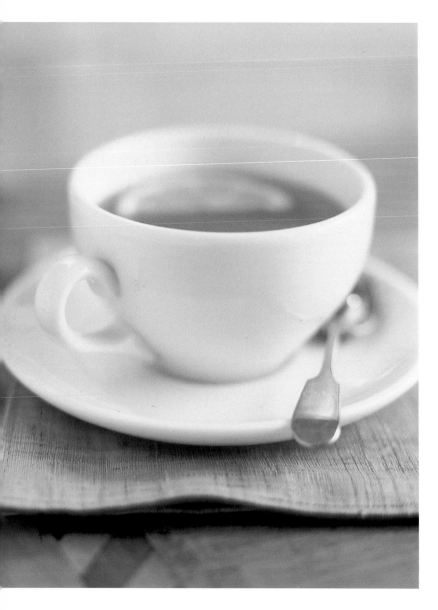

There are a number of health benefits associated with tea, but because of the levels of caffeine it contains, you should drink it in moderation. Also, because it acts as a diuretic, you will need to drink extra water to stay hydrated.

Millions of people drink coffee every day. The caffeine is stimulating to the central nervous system, increasing the heart rate. It can help us feel more awake in the mornings, and improve concentration and alertness. Conversely, if drunk in the evening, the same stimulant can stop us from sleeping as readily, so for a better night's sleep you should avoid drinking coffee in the evenings. However, although caffeine is derived from a naturally occurring plant compound, some people find it has mild addictive properties. Health experts say that despite the health benefits, drinks high in caffeine should be consumed in moderation because they can hamper the absorption of other nutrients such as the B vitamin group, magnesium and zinc. Coffee contains high levels of antioxidants, which the body needs to act in mopping up harmful molecules from the body. Some studies indicate that drinking coffee may reduce the risk of liver and colon cancer, Type 2 diabetes and Parkinson's disease, and it is thought that this benefit can be gained by drinking one or two cups a day.

Tea, and in particular green tea is felt to be even more healthy. The secret of green tea's health benefits lie in the fact that it is rich in polyphenols – potent antioxidants – that are said to be able to inhibit the growth of cancer cells. Also effective in lowering cholesterol, it can help to reduce the likelihood of blood clots, which can lead to heart attacks and stroke. Tea contains less caffeine than coffee, but should still be consumed in moderation.

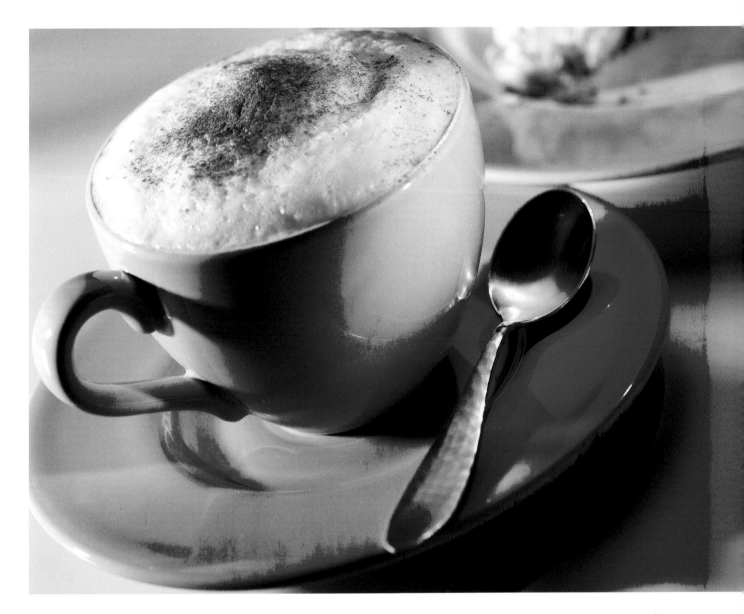

Coffee is high in caffeine, so drink it in moderation. Completely avoid caffeine in the few hours before you go to bed, as it inhibits the body's ability to have restful sleep.

While there are some health benefits to drinking tea and coffee, there are absolutely none in drinking caffeine-fueled soft drinks, which are simply a concoction of sugars or artificial sweeteners, water and chemicals. Tea, coffee and caffeinated soft drinks are all diuretics, meaning that they cause you to urinate more often than usual, and if you drink these beverages you may well need to drink more water than usual to maintain optimum hydration levels.

Tip 70: *Body Mass Index*

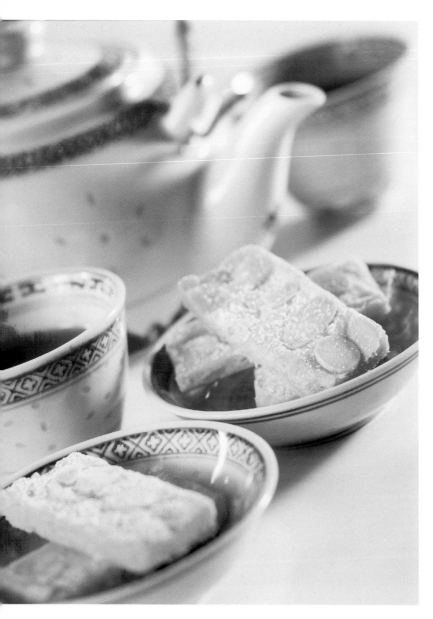

Snack foods such as cookies are high in calories and, along with a sedentary lifestyle, can contribute to a high BMI number.

BMI – or body mass index – is a method of classifying body weight as being underweight, overweight, obese or normal based on a weight and height calculation. It gives an indication of whether your weight is correct for your build and height. It is by no means foolproof, however, as it does not take into account variables, such as individuals with a large muscle mass (muscle weighs more than fat) who may not be overweight, but may weigh more than a healthy BMI indicates. BMI should also not be taken into consideration during pregnancy.

There are plenty of options for those wanting to calculate their BMI – a visit to your doctor, a fitness center, using one of many health Internet sites that will calculate it with information given; (simply fill in your weight and height), or calculate it yourself. To determine your body mass index, use this formula: (weight in pounds) ÷ (height in inches) × 703. So if you weigh 120 pounds and are 5 feet (60 inches) tall, the formula would be: 120÷60÷60 × 703 = 23.4. To calculate in metric the formula is: (weight in kilograms) ÷ (height in meters) ÷ (height in meters).

Experts tend to consider a BMI lower than 20 to be underweight, while BMIs of 20 to 25 are considered healthy. BMIs of 25 to 30 are considered to be overweight, and a BMI of over 30 is very overweight. A high BMI will almost certainly place you at a greater risk of obesity-related diseases, such as heart disease and diabetes. Therefore, if your calculation is very high or very low it is important that you see your doctor for advice on weight management.

If your BMI is very high, your doctor will almost certainly recommend a number of lifestyle changes. As well as eating a healthier diet that is lower in calories, you will be advised to exercise in order to reach a healthier weight for your height.

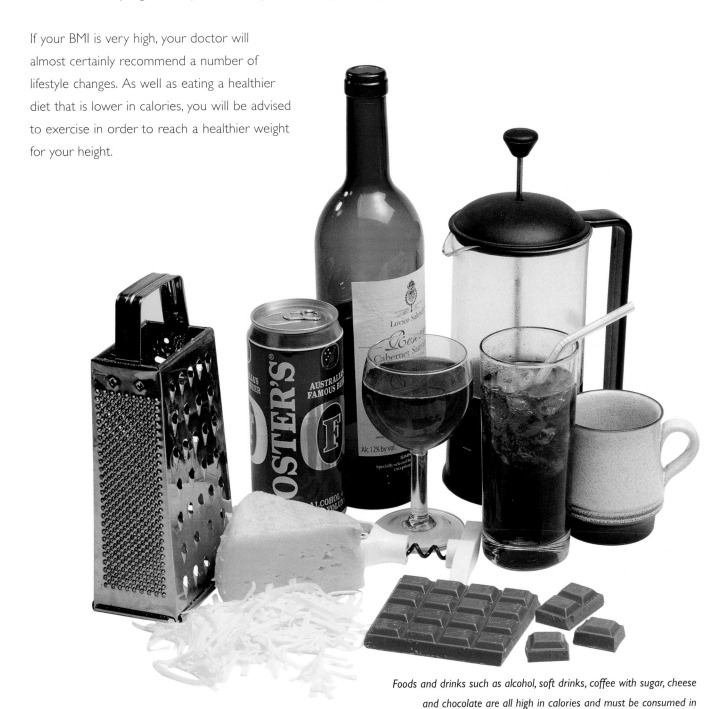

Foods and drinks such as alcohol, soft drinks, coffee with sugar, cheese and chocolate are all high in calories and must be consumed in moderation in order to keep your BMI at acceptable levels.

Tip 71: *GI Diet*

While many new diets or weight-loss techniques are branded as fads, the GI Diet principles have gained in popularity both with dieters and dieticians. It was developed in 1981 by researchers at the University of Toronto, Canada, led by Dr. David Jenkins, a professor of nutrition. Curiously, it did not come to public attention until 2002, when Professor Jennie Brand Miller, of the University of Sydney in Australia, and others, wrote a book called *The New Glucose Revolution*. Within a short time, the idea of the glycemic index, or "GI," had taken the worlds of both nutrition and dieting – which had previously been very much at odds with each other – by storm.

Low-GI foods release sugar slowly into the bloodstream, and therefore are more sustaining than foods with a high GI. High-GI foods leave you with an initial feeling of fullness and a rapid and dramatic rise in blood sugar that is short lived. It is thought that high-GI foods can leave the body feeling low in energy and causes feelings of hunger more quickly, which is likely to be a contributor to weight gain. In order to lose weight using GI principles, foods with a low-GI value provide a steady, balanced supply of energy, giving satisfaction for longer and ensuring that you are less likely to need to snack. Most lists of GI foods (available in health-related books or sourced on the Internet) list foods as low-, medium- or high-GI. Expect to find some surprises on these lists, such as bran flakes rated as high, and milk chocolate rated as low! Many low-GI foods are high in fat, such as chips and chocolate but this doesn't mean you can munch away. GI diets also recommend cutting down on fat, so these foods are still a treat rather than a dietary staple. Following a varied low-GI diet is thought to play a role in preventing or reducing the risk of Type 2 diabetes; and research has shown that low-GI food plans can help to reduce the risk of heart disease by improving the levels of good cholesterol. There are a number of contributing factors in affecting nutritional content and therefore a particular food's GI. Even cooking can make a difference – for example instant oatmeal has a higher GI than plain rolled oats because processing oats creates starch, which enters the bloodstream more quickly. Foods with high fiber content are an integral part of a GI diet as fiber helps to slow down carbohydrate absorption. If you plan to follow a GI diet, you may find it easier at first to consult a dietician or nutritionist who will be able to tailor an eating plan to your specific needs and offer guidance and support while you gain confidence with your weight-loss regime.

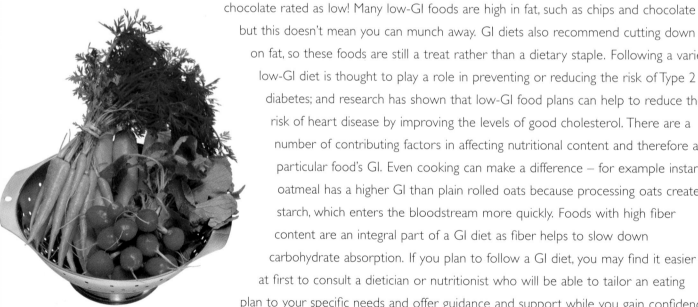

Most vegetables have a low glycemic index, which means their carbohydrates are converted to sugar slowly when they are digested.

Tomatoes have a low-GI rating, but some fruits and vegetables such as potatoes, bananas, melons and sweet corn have a medium rating.

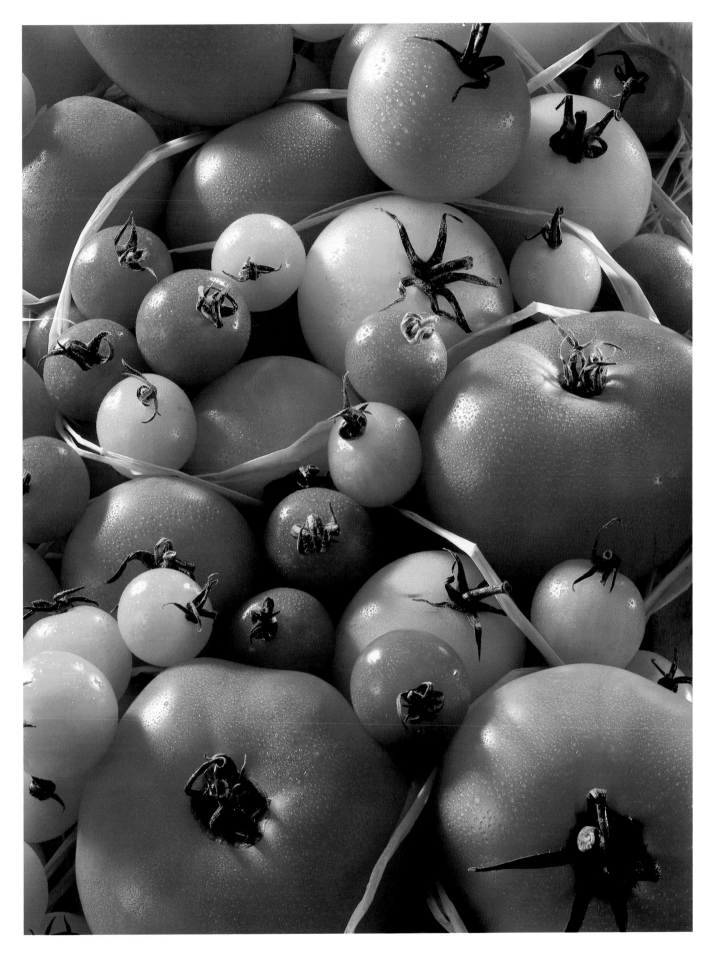

Tip 72: *Obesity*

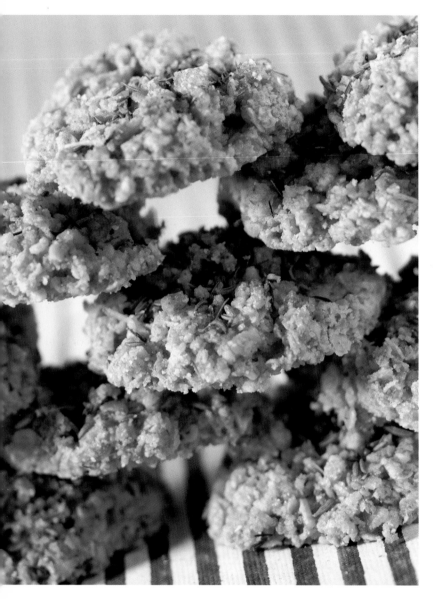

Sweet, high-calorie foods such as cookies are, along with a sedentary lifestyle, a major cause of obesity. Cut back on your intake of sweet, fatty foods in order to keep your weight at a healthy level.

The problem of rising levels of obesity has reached such epic proportions in the developed world that health care organizations are under increasing pressure to curb this modern disease. Even a modest amount of weight loss can reduce health risk levels significantly. Obesity is a major contributor to Type 2 diabetes, heart disease and stroke. It also increases the risk of certain cancers, bone disorders and breathing difficulties. And it is entirely preventable. It is thought that the main causes of obesity are sedentary lifestyles and high-fat foods. Obesity in children is also on the rise thanks to car rides to school, less physical activity within the school day and, of course, TV. As eating habits are formed in childhood, it is very important to teach the value of input versus output – if the intake of calories exceeds the amount lost through exercise, then fat becomes stored in the body. Increase your exercise levels, lower your fat and sugar consumption and watch the weight fall away. Try walking to work, taking a stroll during your lunch hour, walking your kids to school and trying to fit in a swim, gym session or workout at least twice a week. Making it fun will encourage children to see exercise as a normal, healthy and exciting way of life.

Tip 73: *Cravings*

Nearly all of us who have ever tried to diet will have experienced cravings for the food that we have cut out. Cravings are sometimes so strong that even the most strong-willed can cave, and with so much temptation on every shelf, it is not surprising. But there are useful tactics to employ when you are struck with an attack of the "munchies." First, before giving in to any kind of craving, drink a large glass of water or diluted fruit juice. This will give your stomach a feeling of fullness, and very often our bodies misinterpret feelings of thirst for hunger. Deal with hunger first by quenching thirst. Keep healthy snacks on hand and before reaching for a chocolate bar, eat some of the healthier option first. Good healthy snacks include fruits, vegetables, nuts and seeds. If you still experience cravings after drinking fluids and eating a healthy snack, then allow yourself a small amount. Your desire to eat a large amount of whatever you crave will have been significantly reduced. It is also important not to put yourself on a very restrictive diet. The more food items you cut from your eating plan, the more cravings you will have. Remind yourself that small amounts of the food you crave are fine, but keep rigidly to a small portion. Small changes to the way you eat, such as cutting out fatty foods like butter on bread, toast, potatoes or vegetables, will reduce your fat intake without necessarily having a heavy impact on your food consumption or your enjoyment of food.

Distraction is another way to deal with cravings – put on some music or, better still, get out of the house and go for a walk. You may find you feel so much better for having exercised that the craving goes away. It is thought that cravings occur due to blood sugar dips or emotional and hormonal factors, so look for foods that release sugar slowly into the system rather than fast sugary fixes. Low blood sugar is known to cause cravings and blood sugar dips quickly after a

Chocolate's fat and sugar content make it an obvious candidate to cut from your diet, but many people find it almost impossible to give up entirely. Try to reduce the amount you eat, replacing it with healthier alternatives such as fruits and nuts.

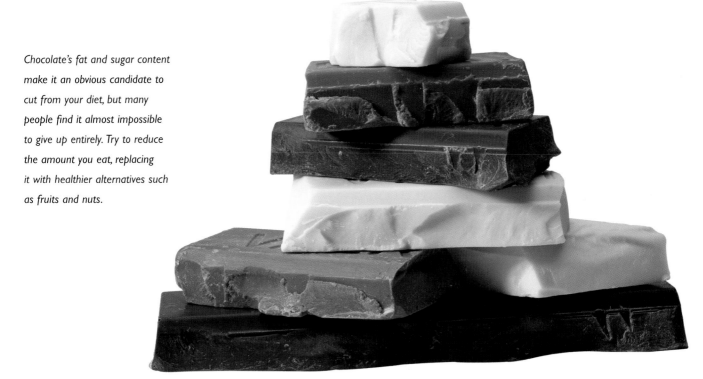

quick sweet fix, making your cravings come back even more regularly and quickly. Depression, stress and boredom are all contributors to eating inappropriate foods, and sweet foods in particular are associated with comfort. Pregnancy or menstruation can also have an effect on the foods we crave (interestingly, men don't have nearly as many food cravings as women). At times when you know you will be vulnerable to cravings, keep healthy snacks and distractions on hand.

It is best to avoid going shopping when you are feeling hungry as you are much more likely to succumb to temptation on an empty stomach. Make sure you eat a healthy meal and drink plenty of water before going shopping for food, and you will find that your willpower is dramatically increased.

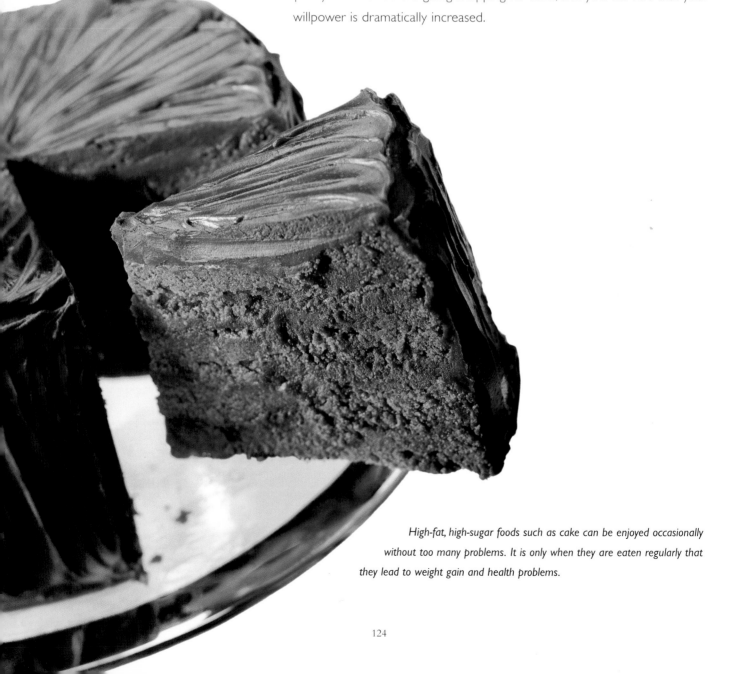

High-fat, high-sugar foods such as cake can be enjoyed occasionally without too many problems. It is only when they are eaten regularly that they lead to weight gain and health problems.

Tip 74: *Staying Slim*

If you are lucky enough to be naturally slim, this is most likely to due to a high metabolic rate. This means that your food is naturally used more quickly in your body. However, many slim women notice that as they approach middle age, weight begins to creep on, particularly around the stomach area. It isn't inevitable that you will gain weight as you age, but you may find it harder to keep your figure trim. Reduced physical activity can play an active part in piling on the pounds, as obviously does increasing the amount you eat. Your metabolism may change as you age, becoming slower the older you get. Bear in mind that menopausal women need 200–400 fewer calories than premenopausal women, so cut your eating accordingly or step up your exercise regime at this time to ward against weight gain. Look for exercise classes geared for older women to find yourself in company with others with a similar goal. Aerobic workouts not only burn fat, but also help to keep bones strong and healthy. Try not to deprive your body of too many regular foods in order to reduce the likelihood of cravings, but revise your expectations of how much food you actually need. Rid yourself of the belief that weight gain is an inevitable part of growiing older; with just a few simple changes to your lifestyle, there is no reason why you should gain weight.

As with any program designed to keep your weight under control, it is essential that you do not deprive yourself of important nutrients. Losing weight is not just about eating less, it is about eating healthier food. Combined with regular exercise, a balanced diet is the healthiest and most sensible way to keep at a healthy weight.

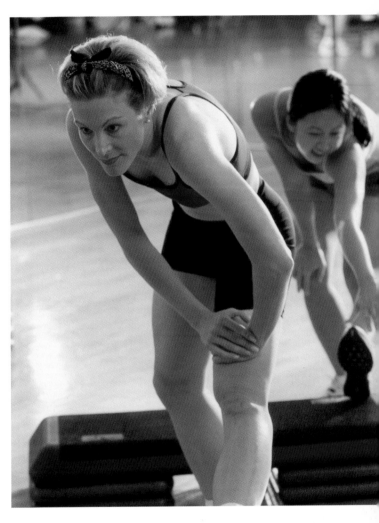

As you get older, your metabolism slows down and it is harder to keep the weight off. Join an exercise class to help you burn off the calories.

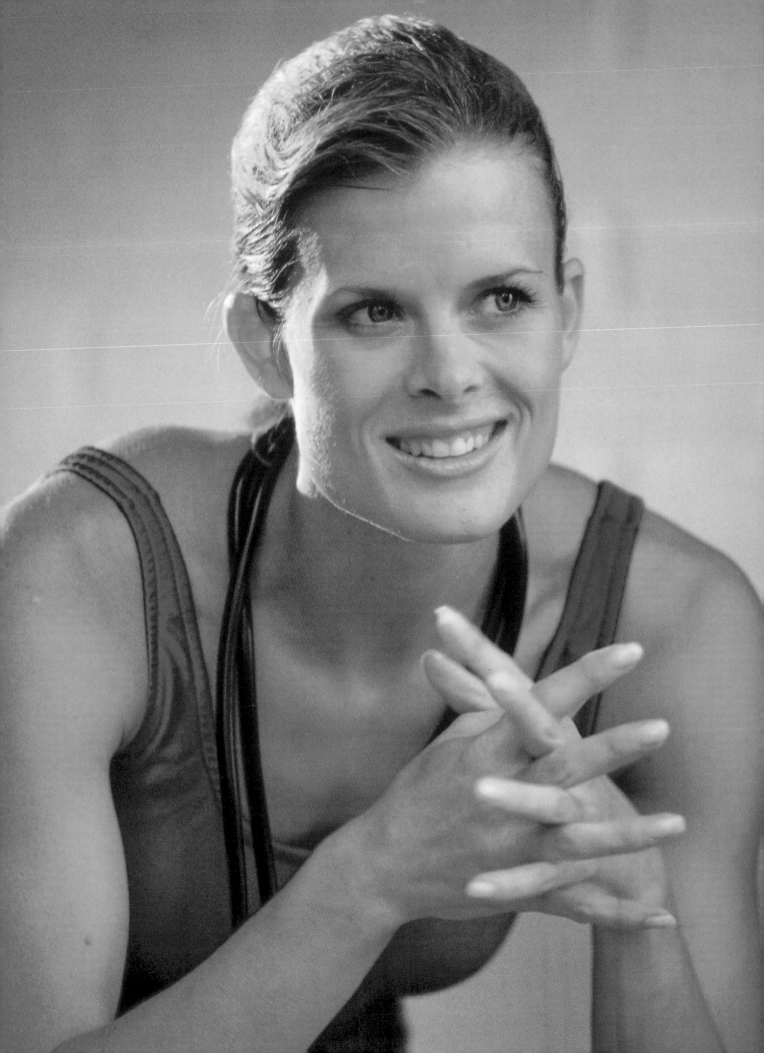

chapter five
FITNESS & HEALTH

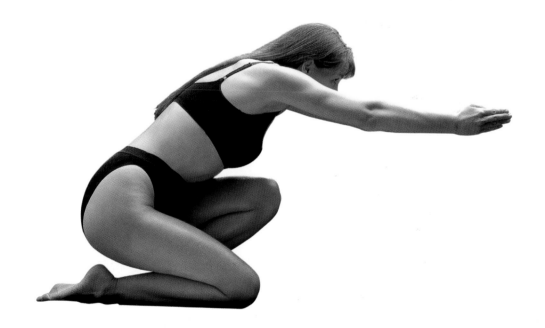

Tip 75: *Regular Exercise*

Today most people do not get as much exercise going about their daily life as they used to – increasingly, jobs and stores are some distance from home so it is impossible to walk to and from them. Added to this, labor-saving devices have taken much of the exertion out of housework, we spend too much of our working lives in front of computers and our leisure time watching TV.

But even though modern life is not always conducive to healthy living, the importance of regular exercise cannot be overstated. And, once you realize just how many antiaging benefits there are to be gained from exercise, you will want to rush out to buy running shoes! There are no age limits to those who can benefit from exercise: young, middle-aged or senior citizens and all the ages in between.

There are so many benefits of regular exercise. Here are just a few:

Heart Strengthening

Remember that the heart is a muscle, and like other muscles in the body, the more you exercise it, the stronger it will be and the more efficiently it will work. Those with strong hearts are less likely to be at risk from heart disease and strokes.

Bone Densifying

As we age, so do our bones, and women in particular are prone to a bone-wasting disease called osteoporosis where the bones literally begin to crumble. But, there is a link between regularly exercising and strong bones – and increasing bone density.

Muscle Building

Muscles gradually begin to lose their mass as we age. Indeed, muscle mass starts to decline beyond the age of 25. Keeping muscles well built and firm will not only keep your overall physique looking great, but will help you burn more calories. It is also thought that keeping your legs and lower back strong can help to reduce the likelihood of back problems in the future.

Stress Busting

Exercising regularly helps your body to cope with day-to-day stress more easily. Exercise releases "feel good" hormones called endorphins that actually help to improve your emotional state and create a sense of well-being. Endorphins are also major players in reducing pain levels.

Weight Reducing

Burning calories through exercise is a surefire way to reduce weight.

Life Enhancing

As well as bringing a sense of well-being, heightening self-esteem and staying healthy, the hard facts are that you actually reduce your risk of dying prematurely by keeping your body physically active.

Health Giving

Regular exercise can decrease cholesterol, increase good cholesterol, reduce heart disease, colon cancer and Type 2 diabetes. It helps to enhance concentration and increase energy levels.

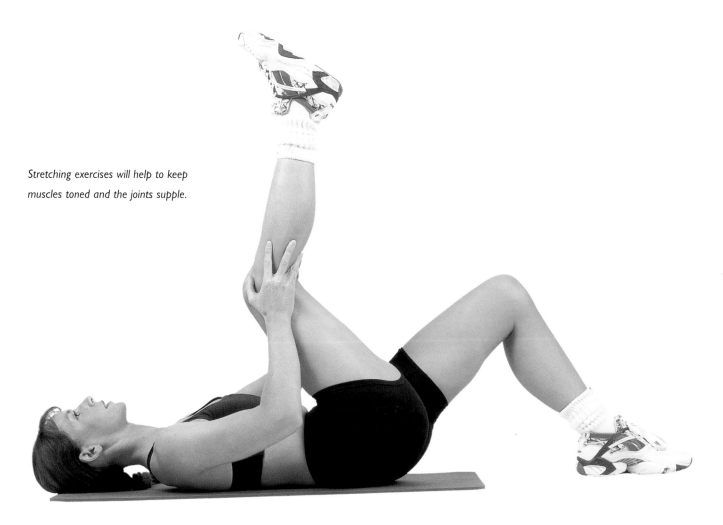

Stretching exercises will help to keep muscles toned and the joints supple.

It is important that you do not push yourself too hard when exercising, especially if you have been living a relatively sedentary lifestyle.

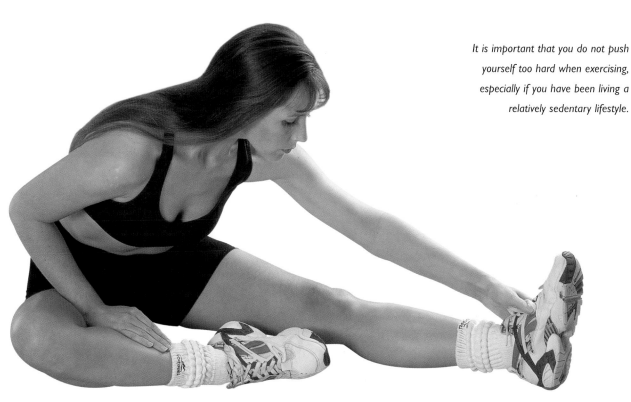

Finding an exercise that you like and you feel able to do at least two or three times a week for between 20 minutes and one hour is important. It is much, much harder to find the motivation to keep active if you don't particularly enjoy what you do. Check out what your local fitness or community centers have to offer. Most will have classes to suit everyone at any life stage, including pregnancy and old age. Keep trying the different types of activities available on offer until you find one that you enjoy; take a friend for support if you feel nervous about trying something for the first time. But don't be confused into thinking that exercise is only for "sporty types." Anything that makes your heart rate increase counts, and you should be mildly out of breath. For example, walking briskly, playing tennis, jogging, cycling or even ballroom dancing are all good ways to exercise. Adding exercise into your life can be easier that you think. Don't let lack of time affect your health. Putting extra effort into normal activities such as heavy housework, gardening or DIY projects can count as long as they leave you out of breath. At work, take the stairs rather than the elevator or escalator at every available opportunity. Park further away from your workplace during daylight hours and enjoy a short walk instead. Get off the bus one or two stops early and walk the rest of the way. Many commuters find the whole drive to work very stressful, try cycling instead, or cycling from the halfway point. You will probably find it's quicker, too!

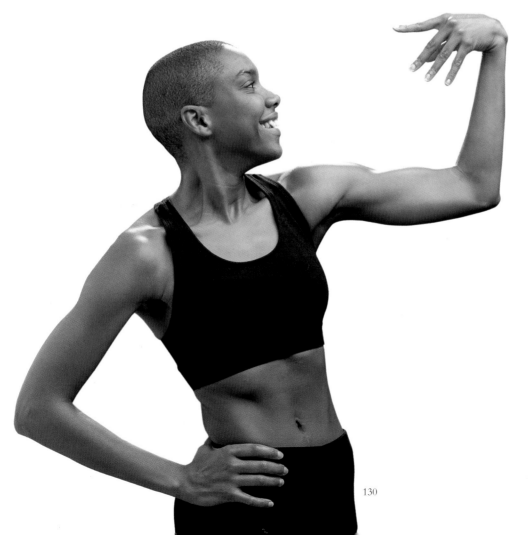

Keeping muscles well built and firm will not only improve your appearance, but will help to burn calories and improve your health.

Experts recommend a walk after your evening meal. Not only does this help you to focus on not overloading on food (knowing you will be walking after the meal) but it gives you a chance to burn off some of what you have just eaten. Showing your children that exercise is just a normal, regular part of life will help encourage them to make good choices in their adult lives. Play outdoor games such as soccer or baseball, go for a family cycle ride or even a family swim to show them that exercise is fun as well as fundamental to your health.

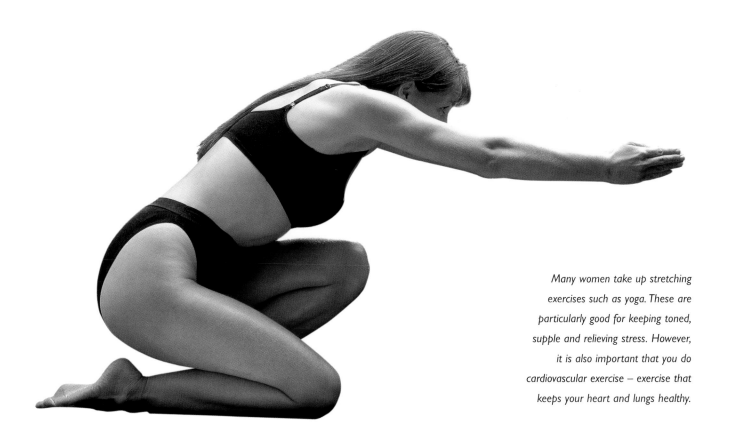

Many women take up stretching exercises such as yoga. These are particularly good for keeping toned, supple and relieving stress. However, it is also important that you do cardiovascular exercise – exercise that keeps your heart and lungs healthy.

Tip 76: *Warming Up & Stretching*

To make sure that exercising is as enjoyable and easy on the body as possible, it is crucial to do a correct warm-up before participating in any sports or workouts. Even the fittest athletes can suffer from discomfort or injury by not warming up sufficiently. Bear in mind that the amount of time spent warming up should be relative to the level of physical activity that you are about to partake. A gentle warm-up before a light swim or walk is adequate, but a more complete warm-up is necessary before more heavy activity like tennis or running. Warming up actually increases your body temperature, which then, in turn, increases the flexibility of your muscles, ligaments, cartilage and tendons by making them loose, supple and ready for safe, comfortable exercising. Without doing a responsible and efficient warm-up, you run the risk of sprains, tears and strains, all of which can be much more painful than their names suggest. A correctly done warm-up will also activate joint fluids (which naturally reduces as we age, making it even more crucial for older people), allowing all joints increased lubrication and less likelihood of rubbing or pain. Warming up prepares your body for more strenuous activity, relaxes the mind and increases your level of safety from injury during your exercise. The warming up and stretching exercises on these pages are not only useful to prepare yourself for more strenuous exercise, they are also beneficial in their own right. Not only will they help to keep the body supple and toned, they will also help you to feel refreshed and relaxed.

A General Warm-up

This should include light activity – for example, a walk before you begin to run or jog – and your fitness level should be taken into account. However you choose to begin your physical activity, the result should be a light sweat and slight loss of breath, and should last between five and ten minutes. Take longer, though, if necessary. By elevating the heart and breathing rate, your blood flow increases to help with the optimum transportation of oxygen around the body. Increasing your muscle and body temperature allows stretching to be more effective.

Stretching

Stretching is one of the most fundamental things we can do with our bodies. It is a basic way of becoming aware of our muscles, bones and skin. We are all aware of our bodies, and may enjoy mental and physical challenges that take our bodies to the limit. Throughout the world there are many exercise disciplines to help us become more in tune with and gain more control over our bodies. Yoga, tai chi, Pilates, ballet, soccer, basketball, running and many more all involve an element of stretching, and conversely our performance in these will be enhanced by stretching exercises.

Stretching involves putting the body into a position that stretches or causes tension in particular muscles or muscle groups. Gentle stretching is beneficial for general flexibility, particularly in older people whose flexibility has decreased

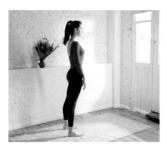

1. Begin by standing with your feet parallel and about shoulder width apart, hands hanging loosely at your sides.

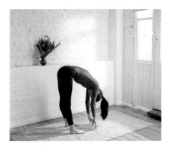

2. Bend forward as far as possible. Relax into the pose then raise your body, bringing your head up first. Take some deep breaths.

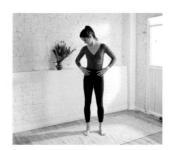

3. With hands on hips, circle your head gently. Do this three times clockwise and three times counterclockwise.

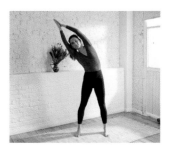

4. Stand with feet slightly wider apart. Put your hands above your head, palms together. Bend gently to the right and relax into the pose.

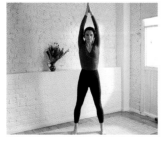

5. Return to upright and hold the pose for a few seconds.

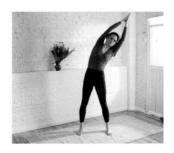

6. Now bend gently to the left, then return to upright before repeating to the right. Do this four times.

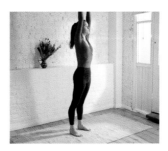

7. Stand with feet parallel and shoulder-width apart. Stretch your arms above your head, making sure you feel the stretch right through your body.

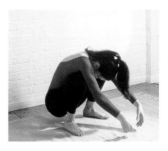

8. Move slowly down into a crouch then gradually stretch up again. Repeat three times.

9. Stand with feet parallel and shoulder-width apart. Let your left hand slide down your leg while the right stretches over your head, pulling your shoulders to the left. Keep your legs and hips still. Repeat three times.

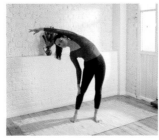

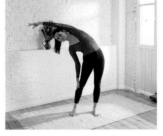

10. Do the same movement with the right hand moving down and the left stretching over your head. Really feel and enjoy the stretch through the left side. Again repeat three times.

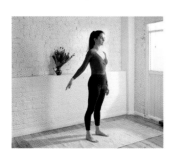

1. Try to set aside 10 minutes in the morning to stretch and warm up your muscles. Swing your right arm backward in a circle. Repeat, swinging each arm forward.

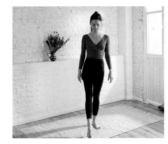

2. Standing the same as in the previous exercises, swing each leg, in turn, backward and forward.

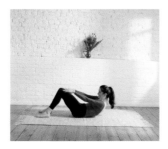

3. Lie down with your legs bent, feet flat on the floor. Slowly raise your head and shoulders until your hands touch your knees. Lower yourself gently and repeat five times.

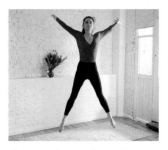

4. Jog on the spot for a minute or so then clap your hands and jump out into a star shape. Repeat several times. What better way to greet the day!

over the years, reduces the likelihood of a strain injury and should last between five and ten minutes. To effectively stretch, put your muscles under tension; slowly increase the level of tension, maintain the position to allow the tendons to lengthen, and then relax. Repeat as often as necessary to feel fully flexible. Never be tempted to miss out on a stretch; lengthened muscles and tendons give your limbs a greater movement range, important in the prevention of injury.

Please do not underestimate the power of stretching and its benefits. Many small injuries are caused by the body's inflexibility. Flexibility also decreases as we age. Therefore, by stretching regularly, we can keep the aging process at bay and enjoy a better quality of life as we get older.

The most effective method of stretching for warming up and cooling down before and after exercise is what is known as static stretching. This involves the gradual stretching of a muscle and does not involve any sudden or jerking movements.

Sports Warm-up

After the initial two parts of a warm-up, those participating in a particular sport should continue on with warming up by more vigorous activity in keeping with the sport's requirements. Adapting your sport warm-up is simple. For example, a sports warm-up for basketball should include more vigorous shoulder and arm movements – arm swings – as these are parts of the body that will be used over and over during a game and not specifically targeted in the first parts of your warm-up.

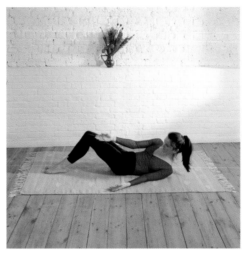

1. To unwind at the end of the day is an ideal form of exercise. Lie on the floor with legs bent and feet flat on the ground. Roll gently from side to side. Let your left hand come over to the right side of your knees. Repeat several times on both sides.

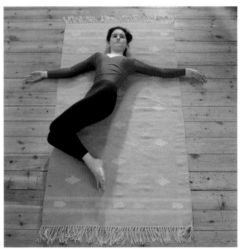

2. Lie on the floor with legs and feet flat to the ground. Spread your arms wide. Let your legs fall over to the right. Feel the stretch then center them and let them fall to the left. Repeat several times.

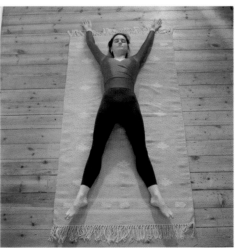

3. Lie on your back and stretch your hands above your head. Feel the stretch right through your body from fingertips to toes.

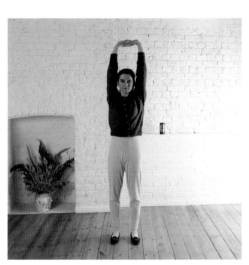

1. Don't forget to stand up and stretch during the day at work, at home or on a long plane or train journey. Stand with feet parallel and shoulder-width apart. Interlock your fingers in front of you and raise your arms, turning the palms upward.

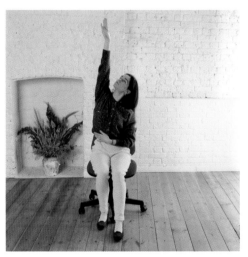

2. Stretch up your left arm as high as you can. Stretch the whole left side right up to your fingertips. Repeat on the right side. If there's room, stretch each leg, in turn out in front of you. Stretch right to the tip of the big toe. Repeat as often as you like.

Sometimes known as dynamic stretches, these are usually more appropriate for serious athletes as there is a degree of risk of injury. Intense stretching uses gentle, but controlled force to move a body part past its normal range of movement. You should have good flexibility before attempting to do this, and to be safe, it should be done under supervision in an exercise class or with a sports trainer where the techniques can be shown properly and adapted to your particular needs.

Remember, even if you are not going to participate in a sport, stretching is a beneficial activity in its own right. Try to get into a routine of stretching regularly.

Tip *77*: *Aerobic Exercise*

Aerobic exercise is commonly thought to be far more technical than it actually is. Aerobic exercise is simply any type of movement that gets your heart pumping or increases your intake of oxygen. While performing aerobic exercise, the body is repeatedly moving, and in doing so, exercises large muscle groups in the legs, arms and hips. Your aerobic fitness is judged by how well your heart, lungs and blood vessels deliver fuel to your body during physical movement. You should aim to sweat lightly and be slightly out of breath to ensure that exercise is aerobic. While exercising aerobically, your blood moves faster around your body to produce more oxygen and energy to sustain the movements. This is great for the heart, which of course has to work harder to get the blood pumping, and each time it beats harder, it is becoming gradually stronger. It is normal to take deep breaths during aerobic exercise, and this in itself helps you take in more oxygen. Lower intensity activities like walking, running, swimming or cycling actually require a great deal of oxygen to provide the energy needed to prolong them. While you may find it tiring at the time, in the long run aerobic exercise can dramatically improve your stamina, allowing you to exercise longer and better in the future. Aerobic exercise can help to rid your body of excess waste products, such as lactic acid, by stimulating the muscle capillaries, and ward off viral infections by activating the immune system. Not surprisingly then, aerobic classes are very popular at gyms, and the benefit of attending a class is that the instructor is trained to get the maximum workout from your body for the maximum gain in terms of health. Usually these classes will incorporate a full body workout, including toning and muscle firming exercises, too. Anyone who is a beginner to aerobics should seek professional advice from a qualified aerobics instructor.

It is a common misconception that those who have suffered a heart attack should avoid all exercise. In fact, exercising aerobically can prevent a second attack from ever occurring, but of course, you must seek professional advice before embarking on exercise. Likewise, if you have limited mobility or ability, it is important to speak with your doctor first. But remember, there are no limitations that won't benefit from aerobic exercise. For most people, 30 minutes of aerobic exercise a day is adequate and is the right amount of time to begin to see improvements in fitness within a few weeks.

Aerobic sports such as badminton, tennis, swimming or running are a great way to improve the health of your heart and lungs, as well as toning up and losing weight.

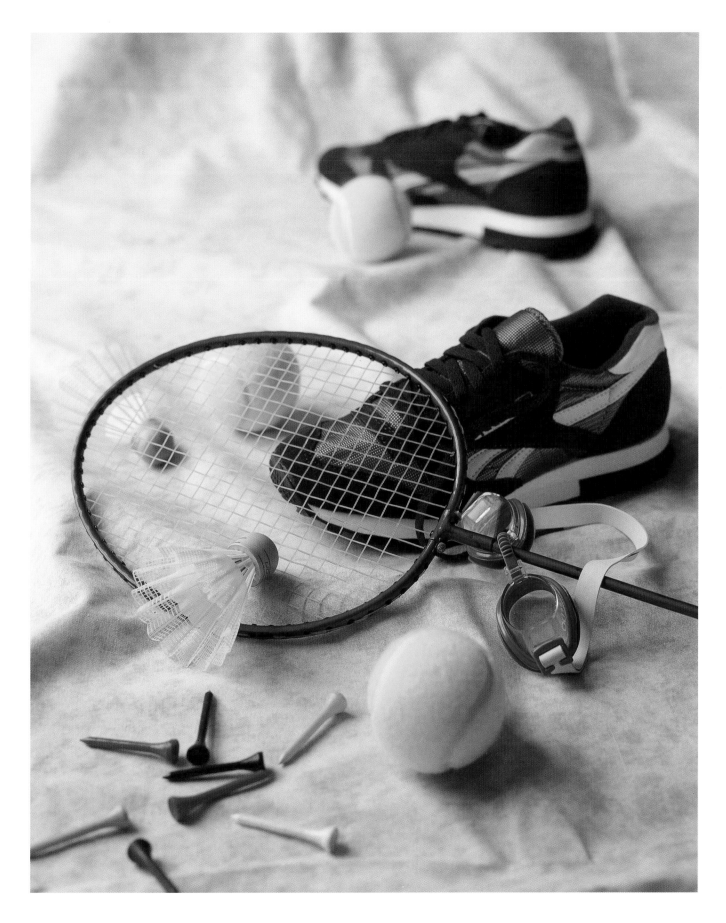

Tip 78: *Anaerobic Exercise*

Anaerobic exercise, essential for muscle definition and strength building, differs from aerobic exercise in the way we use our oxygen. Anaerobic means "without oxygen"; aerobic means "with oxygen." Anaerobic exercise means moving at a faster pace or using greater amounts of energy. Usually this is put into practice with higher intensity and shorter duration bursts, and it helps to burn fat. Anaerobic exercise is not suitable for everyone, particularly those with an illness or heart condition, and is more appropriate for those with a higher fitness level looking to bulk up muscles, although any good fitness routine will use a proportion of both anaerobic and aerobic exercise. Heavy weightlifting, sprinting (rather than running) and jumping are all anaerobic, and they are high producers of a substance called lactic acid. Lactic acid contributes to muscle fatigue, which means that by their very nature, anaerobic exercises cannot last long before a recovery time is needed. Although experts say that anaerobic exercise burns fewer calories overall, it is better at building strength and muscle mass, while at the same time having benefits to the heart and lungs. A person with higher muscle mass is more able to become leaner and lose weight because muscle exercises use a larger amount of calories. Those who are anaerobically fit are able to have a higher calorie consumption, an increased metabolism (meaning that they burn their calorie intake more quickly) and are able to have shorter and more effective workouts. Anaerobic exercise should be done initially with a qualified instructor or trainer as there is a higher risk of injury if not done correctly. The types of anaerobic exercise you should be aiming to do include bench presses, arm curls and weight training, stomach (or ab) crunches. It's also important to vary your routine; muscles become used to routine, and the same number of crunches becomes less effective over time. Anaerobic exercise is one of the few forms in which "working to failure" is acceptable! This approach is often used by athletes or weightlifters where they continue to exercise or lift until they are unable to do one more repetition. Initially you may find that you can only exercise anaerobically for a very short period of time before your muscles become tired. But over time your level of ability will increase, as will your muscle-building and calorie-burning abilities.

Naturally, with high-intensity activities such as weight training, there are a number of health and safety issues to consider. Always seek the advice from a professional at a reputable gym before embarking on this kind of exercise.

A high intensity activity such as weight training is perfect for converting fat into muscle, but it is not suitable for everyone and you should always seek professional advice before taking part in this kind of activity.

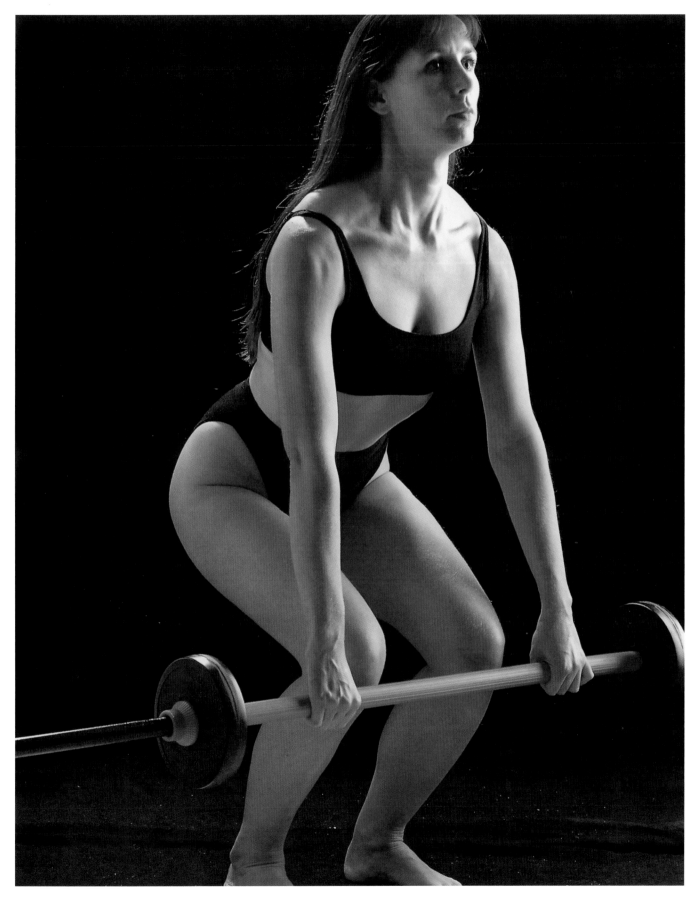

Tip 79: *When to Stop*

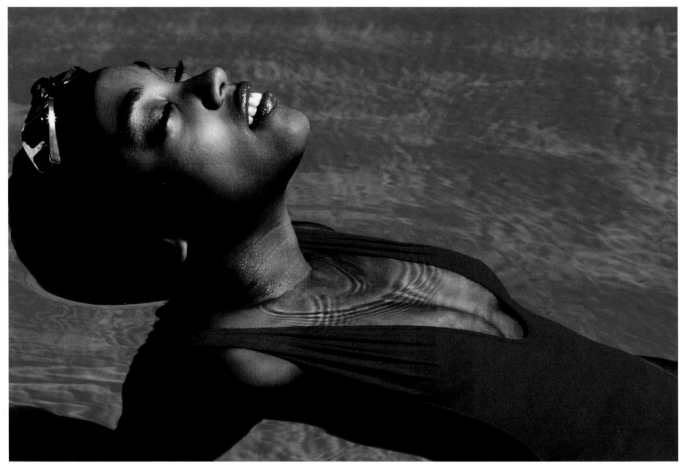

Exercise can become addictive and some people get hooked on it. While too much exercise is better than too little, it is important that you do not push yourself too hard, especially if you are feeling under the weather. If you feel that you may be overdoing things, try taking a break from your usual exercise regime and try a more relaxing activity such as swimming instead.

Hardy athletes positively recommend exercise to work a cold through the system. However, for the rest of us, if you feel under the weather, be sensible. Instead of a run, try a walk, and if you aren't up to a walk, don't feel guilty. If you are a regular exerciser, your body is probably repairing itself well and quickly anyway, so all your good work is paying off as you recuperate. Ease yourself back into exercise gently as soon as you feel better. Knowing when to stop is important, however. A few people find they get such a rush from exercise – euphoria, even, from the endorphins released into the body – that they push themselves too far. At best this can lead to muscle strain, at worst, it can lead to serious injury and exhaustion. If you feel yourself becoming addicted to the rush, try a different, more relaxing form of exercise, such as swimming, for a while. While exercising, if any muscles feel painful or awkward, slow down and do something else that places less pressure on those places for a while. If the pain continues, consult a doctor and leave your workout for the day. It goes without saying that any chest pains, nausea or dizziness could be a sign of something much more serious, so stop immediately and see your doctor.

Tip 80: *Dehydration*

Serious dehydration can be very unpleasant indeed, and can happen surprisingly quickly, particularly in hot climates. First signs of dehydration include increased thirst, a dry and sticky mouth and lightheadedness. The color of your urine is also a strong indicator as to whether you have enough fluids in your body – a strong, dark color is a warning signal for you to drink more, as a healthy color is light and almost as transparent as water. No matter what exercise you choose to do, always have a bottle of water on hand. Depending on how long you want to exercise for, and the conditions in which you are exercising, take an adequate amount. When running or jogging, choose a route where you know you can stock up on more water if the need arises, and always take more than you estimate you will need. Drink plenty of water before you begin exercising and stay topped up all the way through. Sweating, the body's natural way of cooling down, robs you of water and essential minerals. If you do become dehydrated or suffer any symptoms of dehydration, you must stop exercising immediately and drink a sports drink or use rehydration salts (these are available at the drug store and are usually given for diarrhea). Nonetheless, they replace vital salts and minerals, and can aid a quick recovery.

You should really try to avoid feeling thirsty, as it is a sign that you have gone too long without fluids. Get into a good habit of drinking regularly and you should never feel thirsty.

About 70 percent of your body is water; it is in your bones, blood and every cell. We lose over half a gallon (2.5 L) of water a day in sweat, urine and other waste products, so it is important to replenish this, especially if you are losing extra water through exercise.

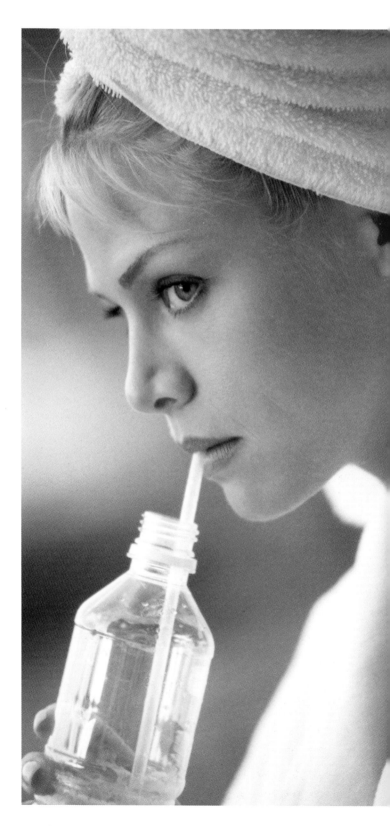

Tip 81: *Eating & Exercising*

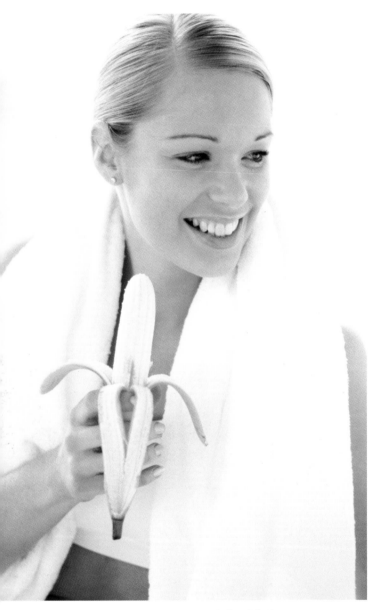

While there are some advantages to working out on an empty stomach, such as the ability to burn more calories, this approach has to be treated with extreme caution. Any existing illnesses, such as diabetes, low blood pressure problems or high and low blood sugar levels can be exacerbated by not fueling properly before training, so if you are considering exercising on an empty stomach be sure to consult your doctor before doing so. Experts recommend that if you do exercise before eating, it should be early in the morning when your body still has some reserves from your evening meal the night before, and it should not exceed 30 minutes. The danger is that without enough food to fuel more than 30 minutes of basic aerobic exercise, such as jogging or running, the body naturally begins to use muscle as an energy source instead. Among other complications, this can lead to dehydration and dizziness. At the other end of the scale, it is important not to overeat before exercise. During light exercise, the body is able to continue digesting food, but with more intense activity the blood supply to the stomach is reduced as it tries to feed the muscles being worked out. Carbohydrates are the key; easily digestable, they keep the blood sugar at a continuous level. Sandwiches (using healthy whole-wheat bread), raisins, bananas and cereal bars are all excellent sources of energy for exercise, as they are packed full of energy-giving carbohydrates.

A banana is the ideal pre-exercise snack. It is full of energy-giving carbohydrates but is light enough not to leave you feeling bloated.

Tip 82: *Pre-exercise Care*

Before rushing into an activity, no matter how busy you are, it is important to complete a thorough warm-up and stretching routine (see pages 132–135) to avoid cramping and injury. It is also a good idea to double check that you have everything you need, including sufficient water, to sustain you during your workout. Don't forget that if you are exercising outdoors, wearing sunscreen will keep you safe from burning, although you may prefer to choose a sun milk as this is lighter on the skin and allows you to sweat more comfortably. Extremities such as your nose, cheekbones and shoulders will need extra sun protection so use a total sunblock on these areas. Also, adequately cover the back of your neck, and wear a hat when it is very sunny to keep safe from sun overexposure. Check your footwear for worn laces or soles. If you have bought new footwear, it is a good idea to break them in gradually rather than start with a long session of exercise, as new footwear can rub and cause blisters and other injuries to the feet. Ensure that you have warm clothing with you for post-exercise cooling – the body, especially if it has become very wet with sweat, can become cool very quickly. Keep away from tea, coffee or carbonated drinks before you work out as these will act to dehydrate you more quickly, and also steer clear of high-sugar foods that will give you an initial energy rush but won't sustain you for long enough.

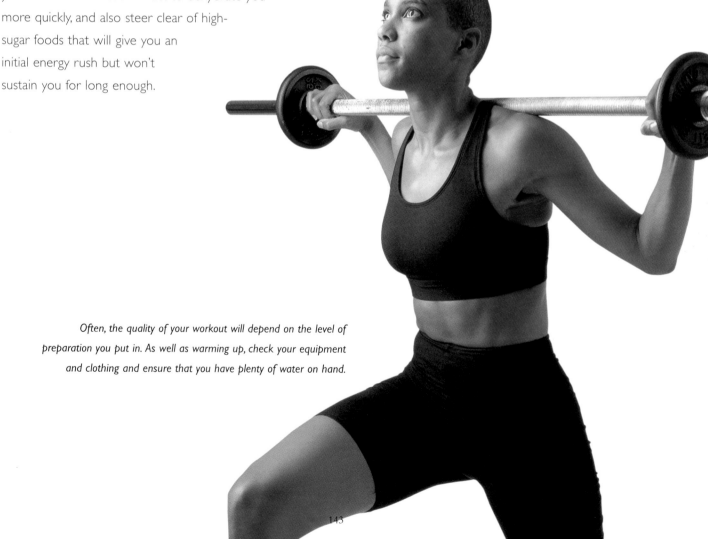

Often, the quality of your workout will depend on the level of preparation you put in. As well as warming up, check your equipment and clothing and ensure that you have plenty of water on hand.

Tip 83: *Wearing the Right Clothing for Exercise*

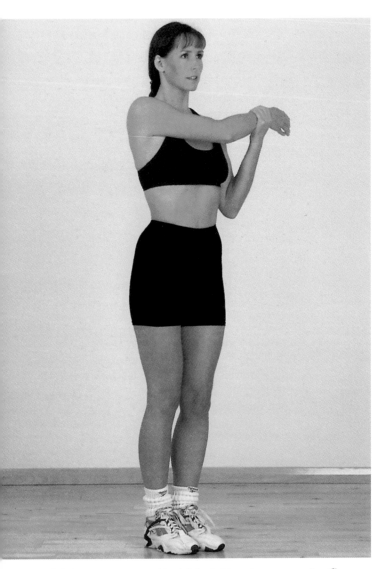

It is important to wear appropriate clothing when you exercise. Choose lightweight garments that allow your skin to "breathe."

Wearing the correct clothing for your chosen exercise will make all the difference to the quality and comfort of your workout. A common misconception is to wear more clothing to allow the body to sweat more, and therefore lose more weight. However, wearing heavy clothing will only help you lose more water, not weight! It also raises the risk of dehydration and overheating. In comfortable or warm weather, wear lightweight clothing that allows your skin to "breathe." While many people opt for cotton, this can actually become wet and heavy, making you more likely to feel uncomfortable and want to stop more quickly. Polypopylene or silk are better at keeping you dry. Technological advances in sportswear mean that there is a huge choice of breathable fabrics designed not to rub or chafe, and to allow you to stay cooler for longer. When exercising in the sun, it is important to wear a hat or visor to avoid heatstroke, and sunglasses to protect your eyes. During colder weather or the winter months, layers work best. Silks and fine wool are good to wear as a first layer as they help to lift sweat away from the body. Choose breatheable materials for your outer layers, and never forget to protect your hands, head and feet from the cold. You will lose body heat very quickly as you sweat, so layers will help you to stay warm during your warm-up and can be removed as you increase your exercise level. Post-exercise, you can cool down very fast, so having another layer to add on top will help stop you from getting cold. For women, it is important to have a correctly fitting bra; there are many sports bras available to buy that reduce movement and therefore any rubbing.

If you are taking part in a sport that involves a lot of time and pressure on your feet, it is absolutely essential that you choose good quality footwear. Not only will good footwear help to keep your feet free from blisters and other injuries, but it will also help to protect your knees and leg muscles. If you are planning to take part in an activity that involves a lot of running, cushioned soles are essential. Footwear should be light but should provide strong and stable support for the foot. Remember to break the shoes in before you embark on a long session of strenuous exercise.

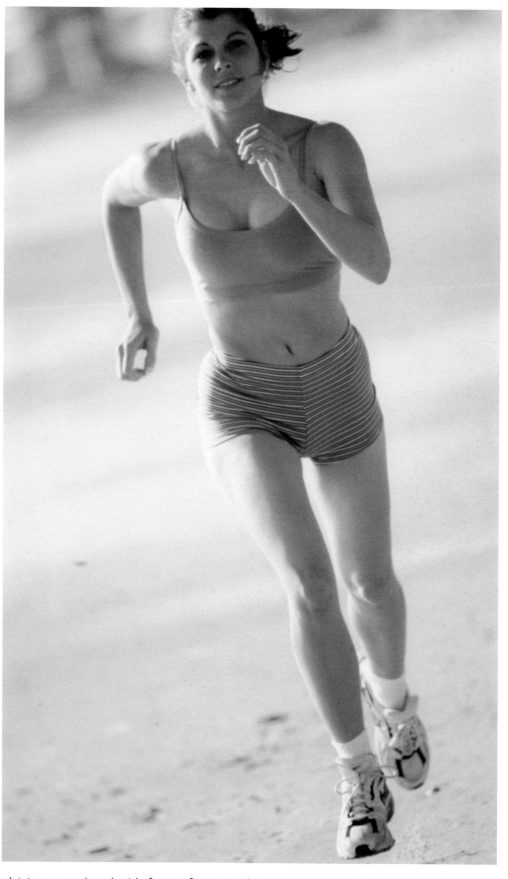

It is important to have the right footwear for any sport, but particularly so for activities such as running that involve a lot of time and pressure on your feet. Soles should be cushioned and the shoe should give your feet firm support.

Tip 84: *Post-workout Care*

If you are taking part in an organized activity or class at your local gym, the instructor will automatically include a "down time," when exercise becomes slower and more gentle, eventually leading to a standstill. It is important that if you are exercising alone, you never just stop. Allow your body to gradually come to a rest. Cooling down after exercising or working out allows your heart and breathing rates to get back to normal and this should be done gradually. It also allows

the body to get rid of any waste products such as lactic acid that have built up in the muscles during activity. Not cooling down properly can have the effect of allowing your blood pressure to drop too fast, making you feel dizzy. Fainting can also occur without an adequate cool-down; blood pools in the larger muscle groups leaving other parts of the body without a good supply. You can ensure an appropriate down time by slowing your activity without completely stopping, and continue this reduced pace for five to ten minutes. Continue to slow gradually, every two minutes, until you feel your heart rate has slowed to near normal. Some people suffer from a post-exercise "low," where the blood sugar dips and they feel faint or weak. Keep a carbohydrate snack on hand, such as a cereal bar, to eat after exercising to combat this. It is best to avoid eating a full meal immediately after exercise, and ideally you should wait at least an hour before doing so. Meals should be high in carbohydrates to replace the lost energy, and high in protein, especially if you are looking to add muscle. You should also continue to drink plenty of water to replace lost body fluids, even if you don't feel thirsty. It's also a good idea to check your feet after exercising, looking for any reddened or warm areas that may turn into blisters. Many athletes stretch after exercising as the muscles are warm and flexible, and although experts recommend this should be done by everyone, it is often ignored. Stretching helps to relax the muscles and bring them back to their resting length. While your muscles are warm they are far more responsive to stretching and less likely to strain. Try to allow at least 10 minutes of stretching

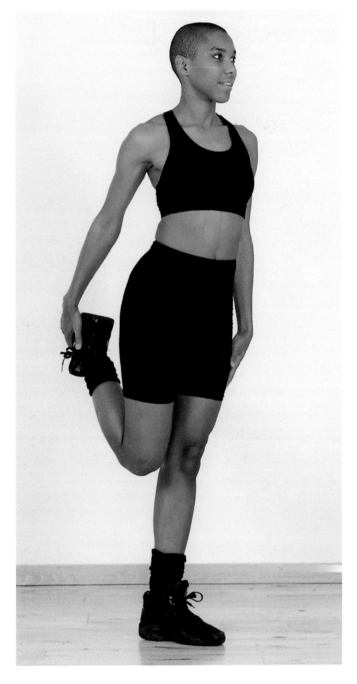

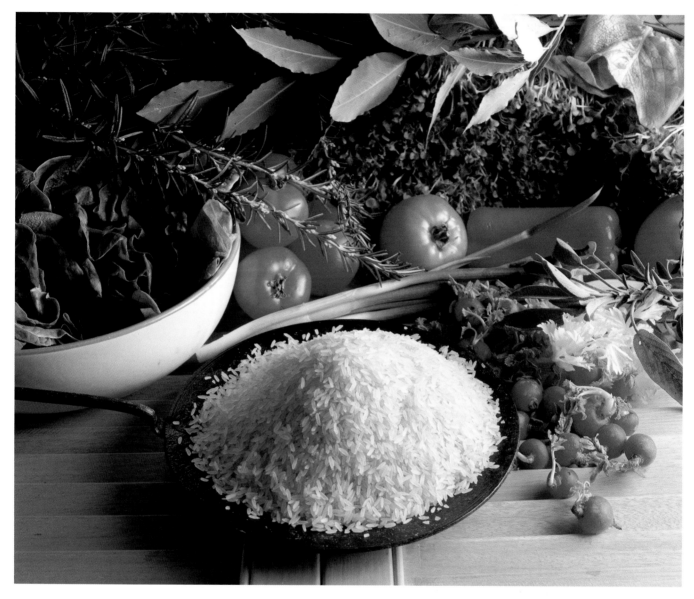

for every hour of exercise you have done. Include all the major muscle groups in your stretch and give them at least 20 to 30 seconds, two or three times. These precious 10 minutes will keep your body in peak condition for your next round of exercise, and significantly reduce the chance of injury.

Rice and pasta are good foods to eat after exercising, as they are high in energy-giving carbohydrates. It is best to wait at least an hour after exercising before you eat a large meal. You can eat a high-energy snack in the meantime.

Stretching muscles after exercise will help to guard against aches and pains the next day and will reduce the chances of sustaining an injury.

Tip 85: *15-Minute Exercise Routine*

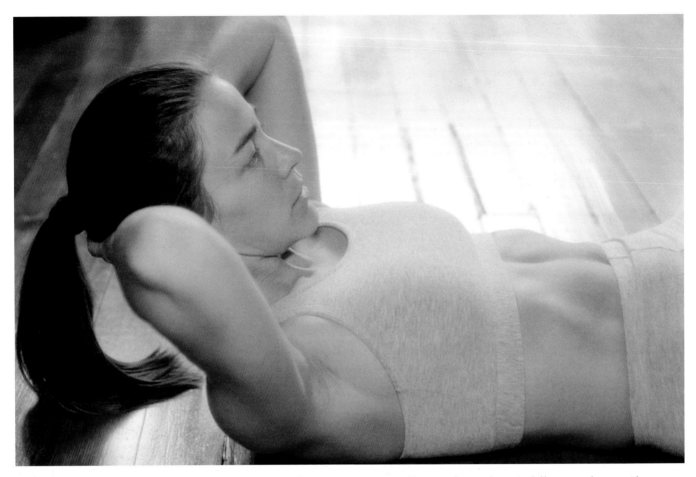

A good way to firm up your stomach muscles is to lie on your back with your knees raised but your feet on the ground. Keep arms by your side or behind your head and raise your shoulder blades off the ground.

Take 15 minutes out of your day to do these gentle toning and stretching exercises. They are good for any time of day, but particularly in the mornings as their gentleness will help to wake up your mind and body. You may like to put on some gentle music and do these exercises on a towel or yoga mat for comfort. Wear comfortable and adequately warm clothing.

1. Lie on your back with arms stretched out on either side. Bring your knees up and turn them to one side, with your head to the other side. Do this 8 to 10 times,

swapping sides each time. Hold for a count of two, and ensure that you go back to the middle position each time (i.e., lying on your back with your knees raised). Make sure that your shoulders are not bending and they remain flat on the floor.

2. Next, lying face-up with your back flat on the floor, raise up your knees, but keep your feet firmly on the ground. With your arms by your side or behind your head, you can lift your shoulder blades off the floor, giving your stomach muscles a gentle workout. Pull in your

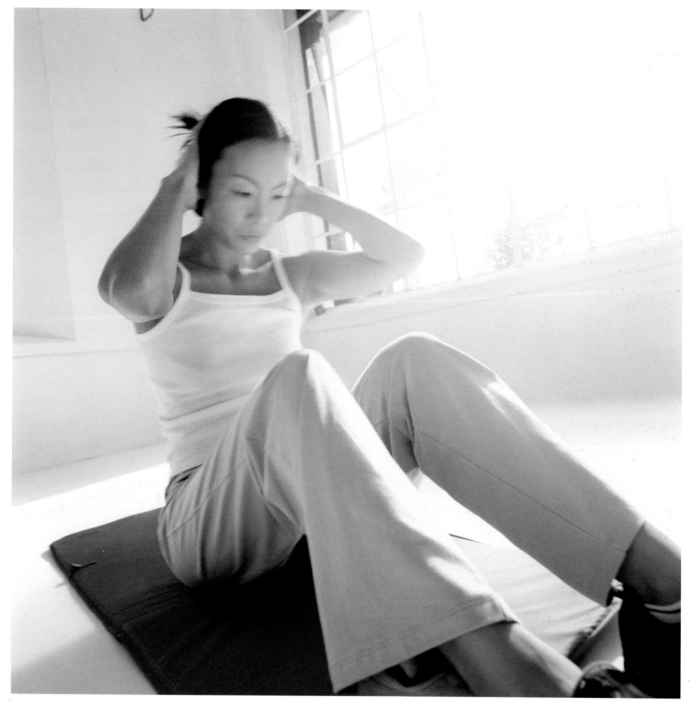

Many people make the mistake of lifting all the way up when they do sit-ups. This is not the most effective way to exercise and can lead to back strain, especially in the lower back.

stomach muscles as you raise, and release them as you release the position. Hold your position for one breath and then gently lower yourself back to the floor. Repeat up to 20 times. The correct technique is shown on the opposite page and the incorrect technique is shown above.

3. Begin this leg-toning exercise by lying face-up on the floor, knees bent with feet on the floor and arms stretched out to the sides on either side of your body. Bring your knees up toward your stomach with your heels together. Try to straighten your knees and extend your legs out pressing the inner part of the thighs close together. Pause for a count of three and bend your knees

back toward your chest. Do this up to 12 times. It is important to keep your back and shoulders flat on the floor to increase the efficiency of this exercise, and you can pull in your stomach muscles to offer more protection to your lower back. If you experience any straining in the backs of your thighs or calves, tone it down a bit. Your flexibility will increase over time. Never push your legs up further than you feel they will comfortably go.

4. Stand up slowly from your lying position on the floor (do this in a couple of stages by sitting first and then moving to a standing position), and put your arms out straight in front of you with your palms facing skyward. Bend your elbows and clench your fists. Raise your right knee to meet your left elbow – don't expect to be able to do this right away! Try the same thing using the opposite limbs. Make sure you keep your back straight and do not overpull – just do what feels comfortable. Aim for 10 to 15 repetitions on each side.

5. To tone your legs, try standing with your feet hip-width apart, and toes pointing forward. Extend your arms out to the front, and with your weight pressing into your heels move up and down as if about to sit in a chair. If you feel unsteady initially with this exercise, hold on to the back of a chair to do your up and down movements. Do this 15 times.

6. For another good toning exercise for the legs and buttocks, stand with feet wide apart and toes pointing outward. With hands rested against the inside of the thighs, move down slowly, ensuring that you keep your back straight. Once you have moved down as far as you can go, hold for five seconds and then slowly move back to the starting position. Do this 15 times. This is demonstrated in the photograph on the opposite page.

7. Standing with your legs apart and feet facing forward, lift one arm behind your head, elbow bent, with fingers facing down your back. Aim to meet this hand with your other arm going up behind your back. Very gently, push for a count of five. Hold one end of a washcloth and raise your arm up, bending your elbow behind your head. Swap arms and repeat. Bend your other arm behind to grasp the washcloth. Pull gently in opposite directions. Hold for five breaths and release. Switch arms; repeat.

Any exercise that involves bending and stretching the legs will be good for toning the thigh and buttock muscles.

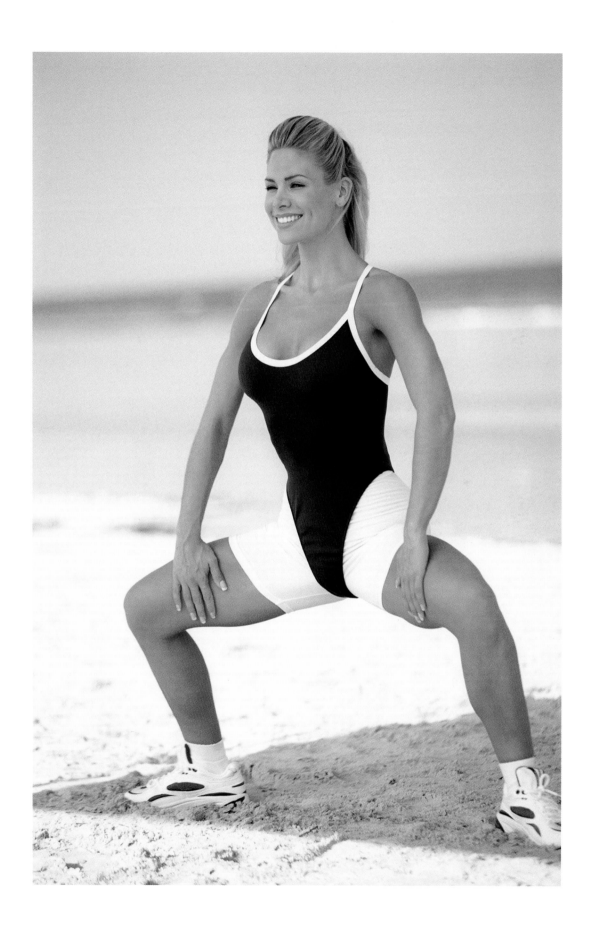

Tip 86: *Exercise for the Elderly*

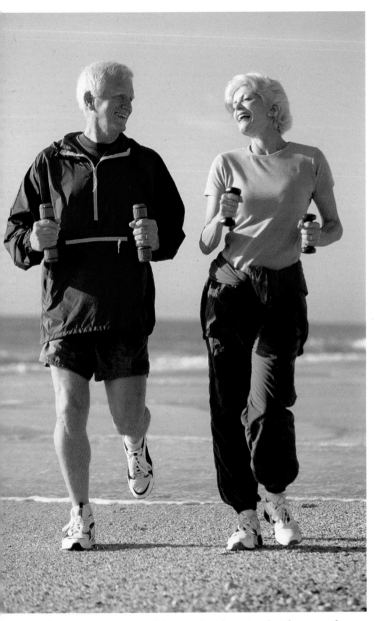

It is never too late to feel the benefits of exercise. But if you are of advanced years, it is important to consult your doctor before taking up strenuous activity, particularly if you suffer from certain health conditions.

Like it or not, for many, growing older means a gradual loss of flexibility, as joints become stiff and painful, lack of strength due to muscle loss and tissue quantity, endurance and stamina, and also balance. None of these things are an inevitability, but how strong and flexible you stay into your old age is very much due to the work you put in regarding exercise. Like everyone else, a range of strength training, aerobic and flexibility exercises will improve your quality of life. No matter how old you are, it is never too late to start! But, before you get started, it is important to see your doctor first to find out if there is anything that you shouldn't be doing. Not all exercise is suitable for conditions such as high blood pressure, arthritis or cardiovascular disease.

When you exercise, wear loose, comfortable clothing and, most importantly, ensure your shoes are well fitting and appropriate for the type of exercise you are doing. Experts recommend 30 minutes a day of aerobic exercise and in particular, walking, swimming or cycling. Ensure that you stretch for at least five minutes prior to any exercise activity, and stretch for another five minutes to cool down, leaving muscles flexible and eased. As well as taking up exercise, make healthy changes to your lifestyle. If you need to go to the corner store, walk or bike there rather than take the car. Use the stairs instead of the elevator. These are very simple measures, but they will make a real difference to your level of fitness. And remember, exercising should be fun – it's not a chore!

Tip 87: *Exercising to Slim Down*

While general aerobic exercise will undoubtedly help you to slim down, you will also achieve a general, rather than specific, all-over toning effect. However, to lose weight through exercise, you must burn fat. Certain areas will take more time to show results than others – notably the stomach, arms and butt. However, as we can't rule where we lose weight from, you could find yourself initially unhappy with the results. Common places that weight disappears from first are the face and breasts. A combination of exercising to slim down and tone appears to give more satisfactory results. The same rules apply when exercising to slim down as do to general weight loss. While exercising will certainly help to burn calories and therefore fat, it doesn't mean you can eat what you like. Low-fat and low-sugar foods are equally important, but one of the many happy by-products of regular exercise is that you may find you can eat more. Combining a healthy diet and exercise will give the best and most healthy results. If exercising is making you more hungry than usual, ensure that you

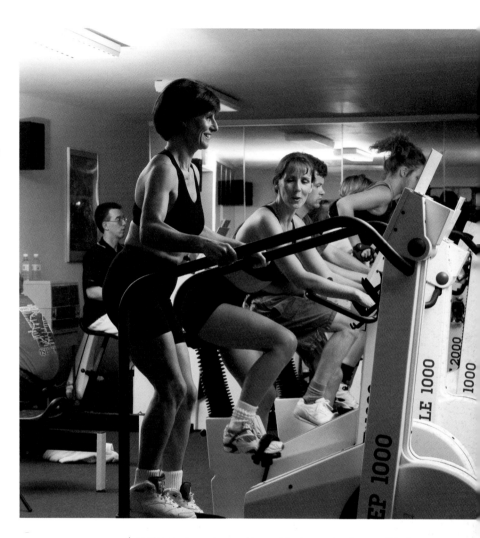

A session on a running machine or bike in your local gym will help you burn off a lot of calories. Remember to drink plenty of fluids and have a healthy snack on hand to boost your energy levels when you finish.

are drinking plenty of water, and stock up on healthy snacks to avoid the temptation to eat quick-fix snacks. If your energy is dwindling, choose a food, such as a banana, which will release sugar and therefore energy back into your system slowly. Do not starve yourself. If you are hungry after exercise it is important that you eat – you don't want to end up fainting because you haven't replaced any of the energy you have just expended. Any program that involves starving your body of adequate amounts of food will not be sustainable in the long run. Exercise should form part of a healthy lifestyle that can be lived and enjoyed long term – it is not about quick results and then reverting back to bad old habits.

Tip 88: *Exercising to Tone*

Toning muscles requires specific exercises targeted at the areas that need to be toned. Toned muscles are larger than un-toned, which means that overconcentrating on an area can lead to bulking up. Unless this is what you want, it is important to control the intensity of toning exercises. Once you have reached a level of toning that you are happy with, then it's strictly maintenance, not further building, that should be concentrated on. Many gyms or local classes focus on a routine of toning exercising, known as body sculpting. This uses a combination of weights and aerobic exercise, and a routine that places the same emphasis on all muscle groups. However, as most women look to sculpt their abdominal muscles, thighs, arms and buttocks, you will find that these areas are concentrated on. However, many experts will say that using old-fashioned techniques, such as sit-ups, bench presses or stomach crunches are absolutely fine – they still work as well as they ever did! If you feel your muscles lack definition after months of hard work, you may need to evaluate your weight and see whether losing a few pounds would show off your muscle tone more. Anaerobic exercise is good for building muscle as short, intense bursts of repetition with weights are a fast and reliable way to increase muscle mass. When exercising to tone, it is imperative that you ensure that the exercises are done correctly. You can – and probably will – hurt yourself if you don't concentrate fully on posture. Pulling in your stomach, for example, helps to support your back. It also makes all the hard work you are putting in to toning up much less effective. One of the most popular parts of the body for toning is the stomach, as this is often shows the most obvious signs of bad eating habits and a lifestyle bereft of exercise. In the perfect abdominal crunch, your back should be flat against the floor – never arched – with knees bent and hands placed behind your head or across your chest. Contract your stomach muscles so you draw your belly button toward your spine, keeping your lower back flat against the floor. Pull in your stomach muscles, bringing your shoulders just a few inches or so off the floor. Breathe in as you come up, and out as you relax back down. Go back down slowly. For more intensity, hold the crunch for a few seconds before you let yourself back down to shoulders on the floor. You should continue this for three to five minutes. The technique is shown on the opposite page. It is always advisable, however, to have a qualified exercise instructor show you exactly what to do, and if you suffer any existing back pain, see your doctor before doing any toning routine.

Remember, you can do as many toning exercises as you like, but you will not see real results unless these are combined with a healthy lifestyle that involves sensible eating habits and cardiovascular exercise.

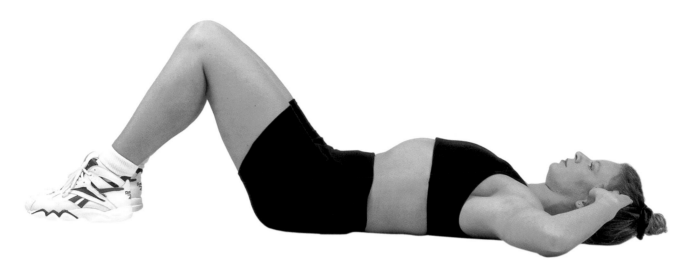

1. Start with your back and feet flat against the floor, with knees bent and hands placed behind your head or across your chest. Contract your stomach muscles so you draw your belly button toward your spine, always keeping your back flat on the floor.

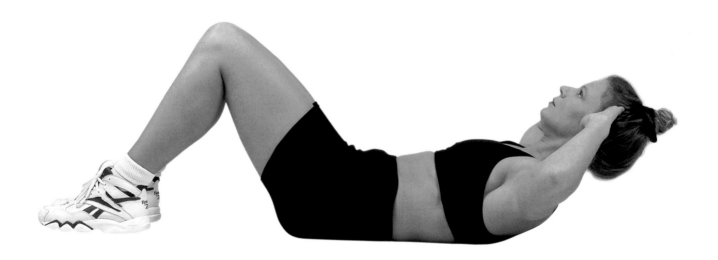

2. Pull in your stomach muscles, bringing your shoulders just a few inches or so off the floor. Breathe in as you come up, and out as you relax back down. For the full effects of this exercise it is important that you go back down in a slow and controlled movement. You should repeat this for three to five minutes.

Tip 89: *Exercise on the Go*

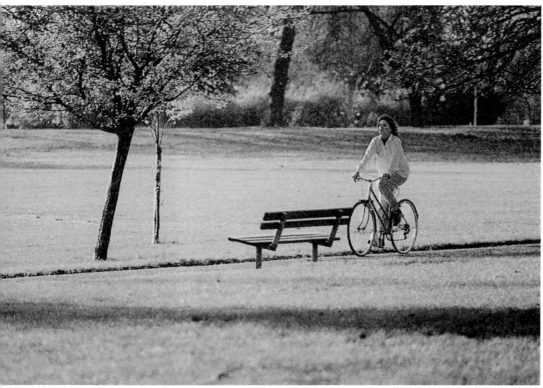

Often, the most effective exercise programs are ones that incorporate healthy activities into the everday patterns of life. A good example of this is walking or cycling to work or the store instead of taking the car.

Without realizing it, you are probably exercising far more than you think! Try to add up the number of times you go up and down stairs in a normal day, and then think about how easily you could do it even more. People actually buy or work out on stair exercise machines when they have a perfectly good set at home! Don't lug a single huge basket of laundry when taking it up in two or three small basket loads will be easier on your back and better on your legs and heart. Likewise, if you have an upstairs bathroom, use that one instead of a downstairs one. When you do your household chores, put music on and get dancing while you vacuum – you'll have fun, exercise and a clean carpet! Leave the car in the garage and walk and cycle more. And if you do have to use your car to go shopping, make sure you use the groceries to do a few arm lifts on the way back into the house; if you have to bend to put groceries into cupboards, bend at the knees and raise yourself slowly to get a great toning action on your upper leg muscles. You can even exercise in the bath, and this is particularly good for the elderly as the weight of the water supports your limbs. To be safe, invest in a rubber bathmat to avoid the chance of slipping, and try some gentle leg lifts. While you sit in the bath, you can try to touch your toes or even do some light sit-ups.

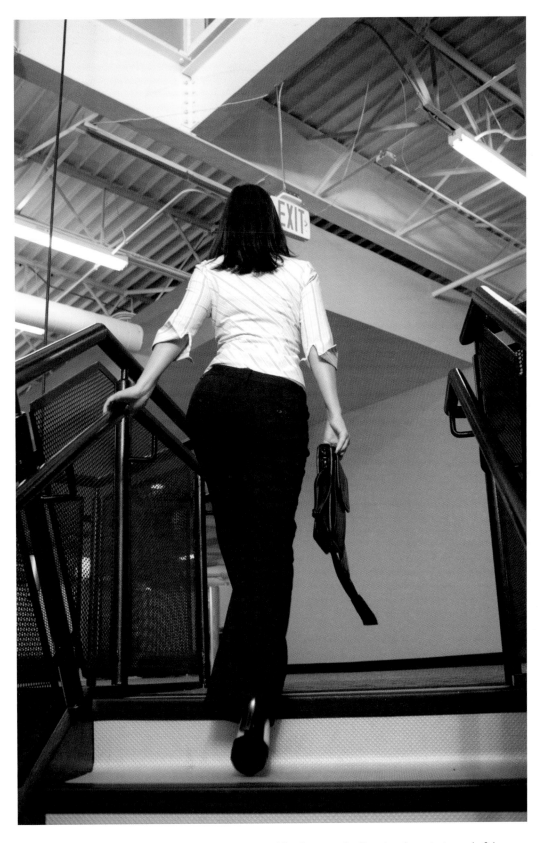

It's amazing what a difference even small changes to your lifestyle can make. Try using the stairs instead of the elevator. It's much healthier, and you'll often find that it's quicker, too!

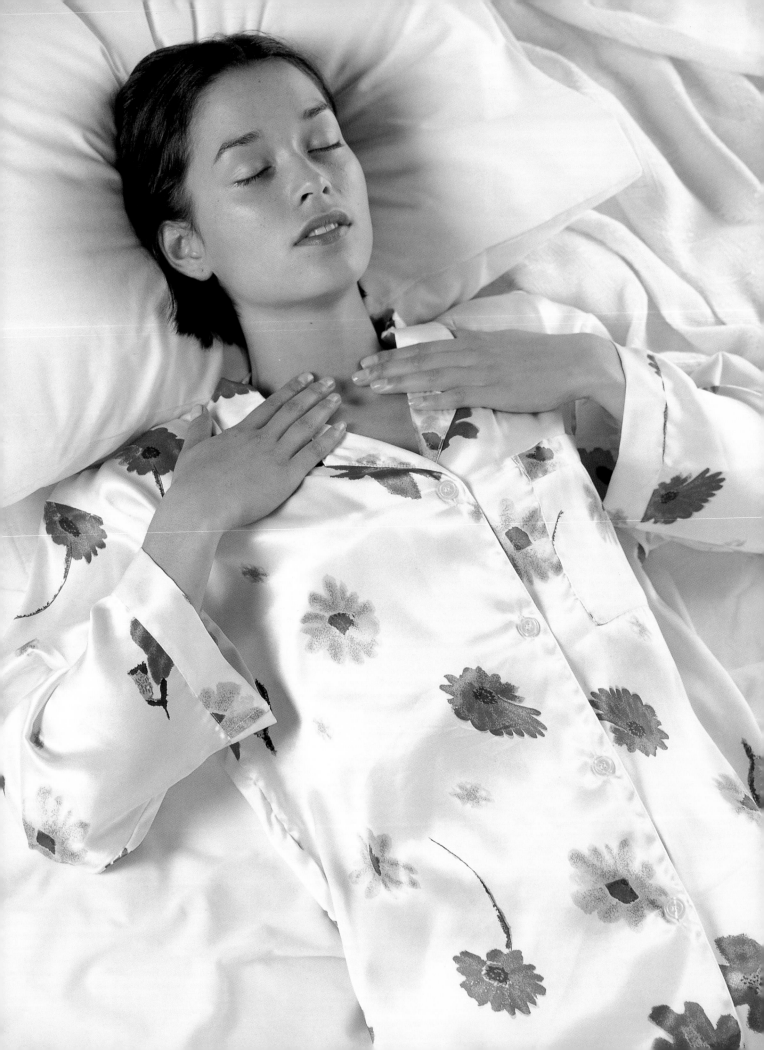

chapter six
BEATING STRESS

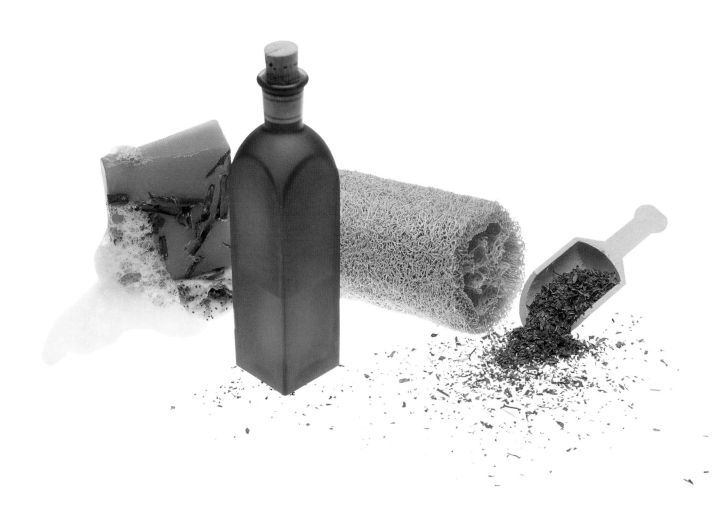

Tip 90: *Time for Yourself*

With today's varied and busy lifestyles, "me" time is rarely just going to fall into your lap. It is something that should be planned for, anticipated and enjoyed because the benefits are abundant. Without space to breathe away from the demands of others, where the time is just for yourself, you will invariably become tired, snappy and lacking in energy or motivation. "Me" time gives a few precious moments to re-evaluate, give yourself a pampering treat or to clear your mind. It isn't selfish to want time to yourself; if anything, the happier you are, the happier others around you tend to be, particularly when it comes to children. Fitting in this time, however, can be difficult, but don't waver! Plan a babysitting swap with a friend, use a babysitter or call in the grandparents so you can get away for quiet time, a massage or just a simple, leisurely stroll. Look at adult education centers where you can join a fun class. Just passing on the responsibility to someone else for an hour while you workout or enjoy a swim is often enough to boost your energy levels and your self-esteem. When things are really tough, however, try giving yourself a 15-minute pampering treatment in the bath, such as a face mask, body scrub or a simple fragranced soap. Choose relaxing bath oils, such as lavender, bergamot or mood-lifting tangerine, to add to the water, and create a relaxing background by lighting a couple of candles and turning out the main lights. Relaxing mood music in the background will really help you to unwind. Ensure that your towels are clean and fluffy. Just the very act of pampering and knowing you are taking care of your skin and body in a way that will benefit is mood-boosting and relaxing. When it seems like there isn't a way to find any time for yourself in the day, try getting up 15 or 20 minutes early. In that time, enjoy the peace and quiet of the household with a warm drink, a short walk if the weather is good, or gentle breathing exercises to prepare you for the day ahead. Try inhaling deeply but gently through your nose and exhaling through your mouth. As you exhale try to "count" the breath out slowly, aiming to make the breath last to a count of 8 to 10.

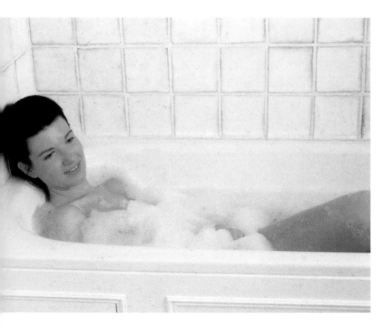

Left: A bath with herbal oils is the perfect way to relax. Lavender, bergamot and tangerine are particularly good oils to choose.

Right: Finding time for a relaxing pursuit like reading isn't always easy, but do try to find a few moments, as time and space to ourselves are essential ingredients of a healthy and satisfying life.

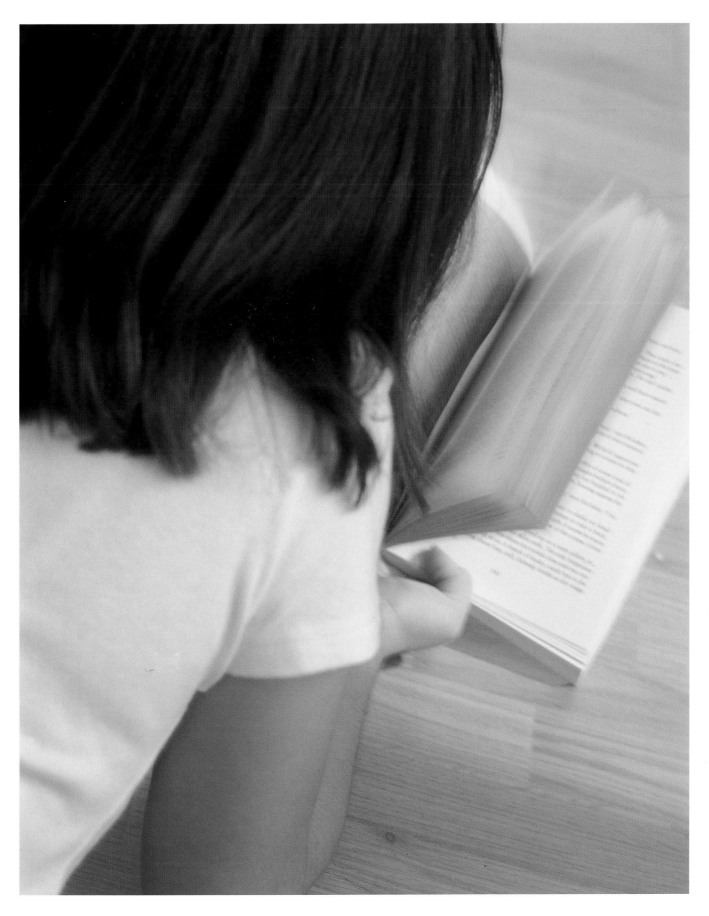

Tip 91: *Relaxing Before You Sleep*

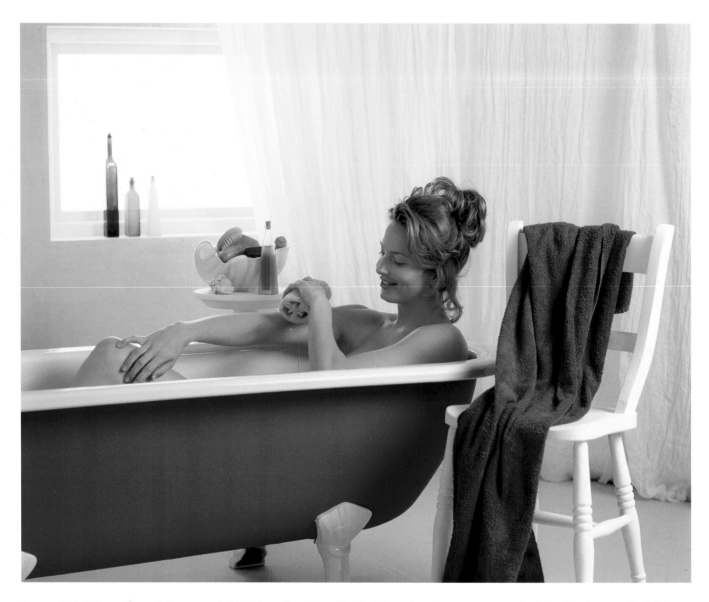

A warm bath is the perfect prelude to a good night's sleep. If you have difficulty falling asleep, the warm water and relaxing time by yourself will help you to unwind and increase the chances of you sleeping well.

Although for many, watching TV can be a relaxing way to end the evening before you go to bed, in fact it can have a negative effect on helping you unwind. While the body relaxes, the brain is working overtime, being stimulated by what you see and hear. Also avoid vigorous exercise right before bed; while it may tire you out, your body won't be ready to sleep until it has had some downtime. Certain foods have an effect on the ability to sleep; some say cheese keeps them awake all night, while others say a banana before bed induces sleep! Certainly, anything with caffeine in it will impact on your ability to sleep, so avoid tea (herbal is fine), coffee and colas for several hours before you want to sleep. Trying to fall

Drinks high in caffeine such as coffee should be avoided a few hours before going to bed, as they will inhibit your ability to sleep.

asleep on a full stomach is uncomfortable, so give your food adequate time to digest before turning in. By listening to relaxing, gentle and quiet music instead of watching TV before bed, you may see a difference in how quickly you are able to fall asleep. There are many ways to help with sleeping, much of it using relaxation techniques to relax both mind and body and allowing you to "switch off" more readily. While some swear by hot milk before bed – and milk has properties that really do aid sleep – others like to use natural methods such as a warm (not hot) bath using essential oils such as chamomile or lavender, to help to soothe them. You can add drops of lavender essential oil to your pillow; the olfactory senses are very powerful, and lavender is known to target parts of the brain via the sense of smell that send signals to relax.

Sleep experts advise that when you are struggling to get to sleep, the worst thing you can do is lie there getting more and more concerned about not going to sleep. It is recommended that you get up and go to a different room to listen to music or read. Go back to bed to try again after 20 minutes or so, keeping to your usual nighttime routine. The temperature of your room can also affect your ability to have quality sleep. A hot, stuffy room is a recipe for disaster regarding sleep, making you sticky and uncomfortable before you even start. On hot nights, a cool shower before bed and a simple electric fan can make all the difference. In fact, "white noise" such as a bedside fan can help some people to drift off. Choose cotton or silk clothing to wear in bed, but make sure your clothing is comfortable and not restrictive in any way. Choose cotton bed sheets that are gentle on the skin, and help to keep you at a comfortable temperature. A cold room, while thought to be "healthier," is no fun to sleep in if you wake up shivering! Take a hot water bottle to bed with you while you wait for your body to naturally conserve heat as you sleep.

Tip **92**: *Bathing, Showering & Spas*

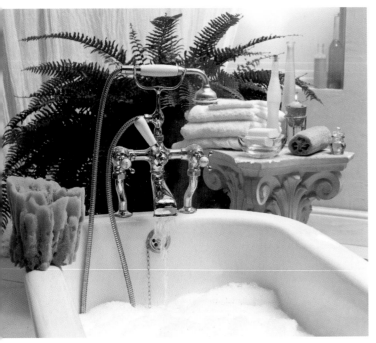

A few well-chosen accessories can add to the pleasure of bathing and make it a blissful as well as a cleansing experience. Develop bathtime rituals that guarantee you the full benefits of bathing.

To think of bathing and showering solely in terms of cleansing the body is to ignore the many ways in which this daily ritual can enhance your well-being. Bathing offers a multitude of benefits. It can be a therapeutic, sensual, calming, invigorating or uplifting experience.

Using water to cleanse, relax or invigorate couldn't be easier and more effective. Bathing rituals are centuries old, where water was used to purify; Cleopatra was believed to have bathed in donkey's milk (which would have had skin softening properties but wouldn't have smelled great), Egyptians used bathing before prayer, while the Greeks used cold showers as a fortifying technique. Ancient and current Japanese bathing rituals are used to bond man and nature. Believe it or not, there is an optimum bathing temperature: 112°F/45°C (for young children it is 100°F/38°C), but how warm or cool you like your soak is a personal choice. However, experts warn against having your bath water too hot as this can lead to blood vessel damage and overheating, and those with high blood pressure should avoid very hot baths.

Bathing can be an intensely therapeutic experience rather than just a cleaning opportunity, so treat it as just that: a chance to release stress and relax. Find time when you are not likely to be disturbed, light scented candles, pick out your favorite book or put on some relaxing music. Use bathing time to treat yourself to beneficial beauty treatments such as a face mask or a body scrub. Water is wonderful for soothing the muscles, easing joint stiffness and helping to reduce aches and pains. Because bathing is such a

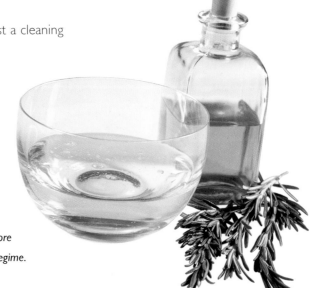

A range of natural oils are available to make the bathing experience even more pleasurable. They not only help you to relax, but also play a role in your beauty regime.

comfortable experience, it is also good for inner well-being; the feeling of warmth and relaxation helps us to feel nurtured and secure. Using water to soothe your mood can be helped by adding essential oils, bubble baths, herbs or salts to the water. If you choose to bathe at bedtime, adding a few drops of lavender essential oil can help to aid sleep and relaxation, as can chamomile and jasmine. Essential oils are thought by practitioners of aromatherpay to have healing effects. In addition to affecting specific organs, essential oils act upon the limbic part of the brain (its most primitive area, which is concerned with emotions). The mental and emotional influence is determined by the oil you choose, so ensure you read the label before adding to your bath. Herbs, which are often used to make essential oils, can have a similarly soothing effect. They can contain complex substances, including essential vitamins, minerals and oils. Adding herbs to your bath is a gentler, less concentrated

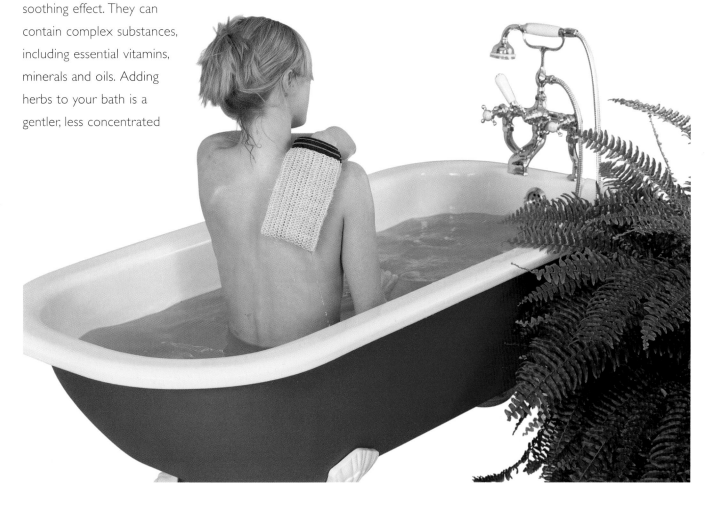

Above: Herbs can have an invigorating effect. They are available in powder form or in the form of essential oils.

Below: Exfoliating gloves can be used to great invigorating effect. The back and the soles of the feet are particularly good places to use them.

In addition to affecting specific organs, it is thought that essential oils act upon the limbic part of the brain, which is concerned with emotions. The mental and emotional influence is determined by the oil you choose, so ensure you read the labels and pick the one that is most appropriate for you.

way of using herbs than eating or drinking them, but can be equally therapeutic. When you add herbs to your bath, they have a twofold effect. They are absorbed by your skin – carrying their active ingredients – but you acquire an added benefit from breathing in their calming vapors. A hardy few are prepared to go for the ultimate in skin toning and invigorating water experiences – the cold bath! Don't, however, do this if you feel under the weather or have any medical contraindications. A cold bath is purely to awaken and revive, and while cold water does have skin toning effects, there are more comfortable ways to do this, such as investing in a good toning lotion! Develop bathtime rituals that guarantee you the full benefits of bathing. Find out how to exfoliate, and what are the most suitable products to use. Discover which bath products are best for your skin, and spend time in the bath to give your hair a transforming treatment. Counter the drying effect of the water with a moisturizing body lotion. Tackle rough skin on areas such as your hands and feet to keep them in perfect condition. Simple techniques, such as scrubbing or brushing your skin before you jump into the bath or shower, not only feel good but are immensely beneficial. Regular exfoliation helps to remove dead particles, leaving the skin softer and smoother. The friction also boosts circulation and unclogs blocked pores, so that skin looks fresher. A wide range of exfoliation equipment is available, from loofahs, brushes and gloves to creams and gels. The act of exfoliating can be very therapeutic, and will help you to look and feel invigorated and fresh.

Showers, on the other hand, tend to be more invigorating and a popular way to help wake up in the mornings. But findings have shown that showering can also help to increase the heart rate and blood flow, improving circulation. Try beginning your shower warm and gradually reducing the temperature to cool for a more refreshing and stimulating experience; this is also a great way to cool down in hot summer months. Exfoliating in the shower is beneficial too and is better than in bath where loosened skin cells stay in the water. Use a salt scrub or a loofah to give your skin a thorough exfoliation but massage in a moisturizer afterward to avoid having your skin feel taut.

If you are lucky enough to have a home spa or a bubble jet bath, this is the perfect opportunity to create a truly relaxing and beautifying treat. The actions of the jets or bubbles is thought to have a benefit in helping cellulite by increasing circulation and lymphatic drainage in stubborn areas such as hips and thighs, which in turn helps to rid the body of toxins. They also act to massage the body, which can be intensely relaxing and soothing, particularly after exercise where you may have a few aches and pains.

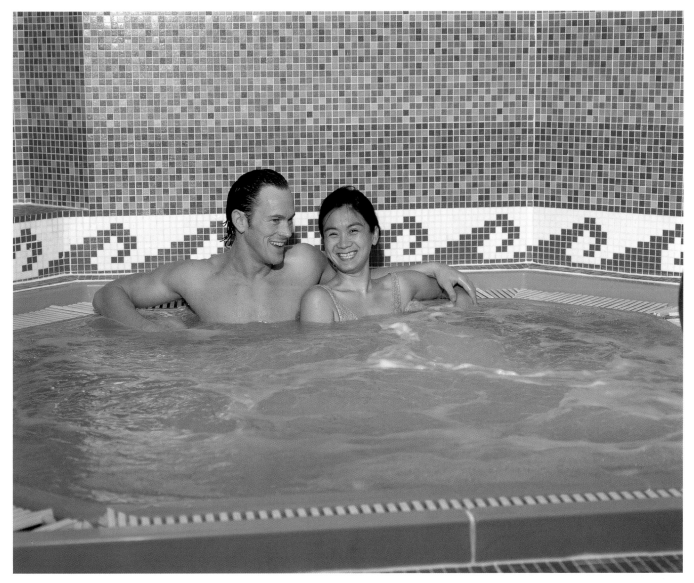

A home spa with a bubble jet facility has a number of health and beauty benefits. The actions of the bubbles help to relax and sooth tired muscles, as well as aiding the control of cellulite by increasing circulation and lymphatic drainage in areas such as the hips and thighs.

Try to maintain good hygiene practices around your bathing areas. Showers, baths and spas are notorious germ traps, particularly if it is a shared facility. You can remove any hard water deposits with a solution of white vinegar and water, and you should always leave your shower door open to allow air to circulate, discouraging the buildup of germs and mildew. Remove any trapped hair from the drain holes, and always wipe down the area with a disinfectant-based cleaning product.

Tip 93: *Massage: Basic Strokes*

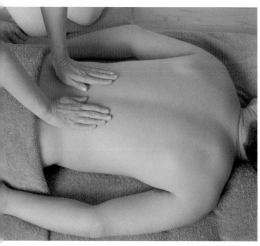

Effleurage is a form of stroking that is particularly good in relieving stress and tension. Using the flat of the hand, the fingers are kept close together, with the fingertips slightly raised so they do not dig into the skin as you stroke.

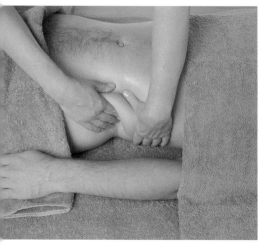

Kneading should be carried out by keeping the fingers straight, lifting the tissue away from the bone in one hand, then passing it over to the other hand, before grasping another handful, as if you were kneading bread.

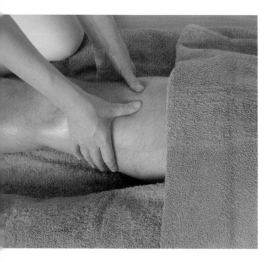

Petrissage comes from the French word Petrir, meaning "to knead." Use the fingers or thumbs to squeeze the soft tissue against the bone beneath in small, circular motions, trapping the skin rather than sliding over it.

Massage is not only an important way of communicating via the sense of touch, but can also help with well-being and relaxation. The human body stores stress, in the neck, back, head and shoulders, and a good massage will help to relieve any tensions in these areas as well as result in an emotional stress release. One of the first rules of massage is to make movements that go with the flow of the body, toward the heart. If you massage the stomach area, this should be done clockwise using a circular motion. You can add aromatherapy oils to your basic massage oil if you prefer, but a good basic oil to use is sweet almond oil. Try to maintain hand to body contact at all times and keep the strokes fluid. Greater pressure can be applied to areas such as the shoulders, back and buttocks, but go gently over bony areas and the stomach. To prepare for massage, ensure that you have soft towels available to lie on, that your room temperature is ambient, draft-free, and the environment quiet and relaxed.

Massage is not just a treat or a whimsy – it really does help you to feel better. Even the most basic massage, done without any training or instruction, helps to stimulate the circulation and dilate the blood vessels. You can see this happening when the area that you massage reddens. The improved blood flow helps to reoxygenate the tissues, bringing nutrients to the site and taking away toxins. It also boosts the lymphatic system and can reduce fluid retention. The heat produced by the massage and the extra blood flow helps to relax muscular tension.

Regular deep-tissue massage can be extremely helpful if you are under stress, particularly if you combine it with the therapeutic properties of sedative aromatherapy oils, which are readily absorbed into the skin during massage.

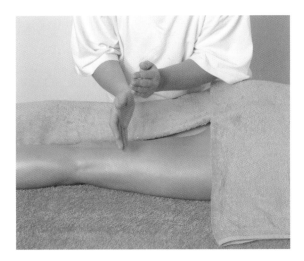

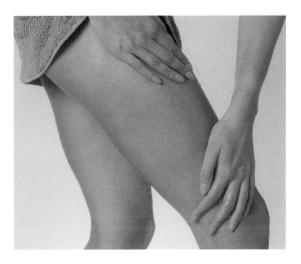

There are several percussive strokes: hacking (pictured above), using the little finger edges of each hand in a smooth, chopping motion; cupping, using curved palms to tap the skin, which creates a mini-vacuum and produces a sound like trotting hooves; and tapotement, a gentle tapping with the fingertips that is useful for the sensitive skin of the face.

Rub the palms quickly over the body, producing heat through friction. For a more pronounced effect, wear a sisal mitten.

If you visit a therapist for your massage, it should comprise some if not all of the movements listed below.

Effleurage

This is a slow, rhythmic stroking and is used to begin and end each massage session. It helps to increase the body's circulation and absorption of the skin softening oils. It is particularly effective at releasing stress and tension.

Kneading

Kneading is an excellent stroke for the fatty areas of the body, such as the thighs and buttocks. It is a very effective way of releasing toxins from these parts of the body. It should never cause any pain, so go slowly and carefully to relieve any knots.

Petrissage

This is another kneading technique, but it is used on less fatty parts of the body where muscle is knotted or tense and the bone is close to the surface.

Percussion

This is a stimulating massage technique that should be performed quickly. It can be used all over the body, but is particularly good for fatty areas such as the hips and thighs.

Friction

This is a fast, but not necessarily hard rubbing movement that helps to increase circulation, so is great for any areas that are cold, such as the hands and feet. This technique is very easy to try on yourself.

Tip 94: *Self-massage & Tension Release*

It isn't always necessary to visit a therapist or rely on someone else for a stress-busting massage. There are many massage techniques that can be applied to oneself that are both effecting and relaxing. A good place to massage yourself is in the bathtub, when your body is warm and the muscles more pliant and receptive.

Feet

Heading from the toes toward the ankles, keep your thumb on the top side of your foot, and have your fingers underneath. Gently draw your fingers up and down the underside of the foot rhythmically (your thumb should be doing the same on the front of the foot), and finish by paying individual attention to each of the toes. Try this sitting with your legs crossed for easy access.

Hands

Fingers are full of nerve endings, so they are particularly sensitive to massage. You may find it helpful to soak them in warm water first before applying oils and beginning to massage. Using stroking movements with your thumb on the palm of your hand at your wrist you can use your other fingers over the top to stroke from your wrist all the way up to the ends of each individual finger. Squeeze each finger and use circular motions over the joints. Do this several times, and swap hands.

Head

This head massage is a great way to relieve stress and tension.

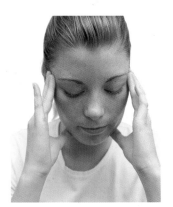

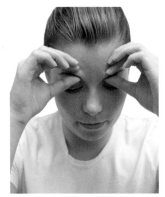

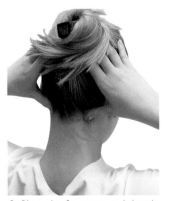

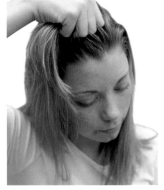

1. Using both hands, one on either side of your face, drag the tips of your middle three fingers down your jaw line from the temples. Brace with thumbs under the jaw.

2. Using thumb and forefinger, squeeze your eyebrows, starting at your nose, moving out toward the temples.

3. Place the fingertips and thumb of each hand on either side of your head behind your ears. Aim to move the skin in small circles across the bone of your scalp, massage the entire scalp.

4. Grasp handfuls of hair near the roots, and tighten your grasp, pulling gently on the roots. Move the handfuls until the whole scalp has been pulled.

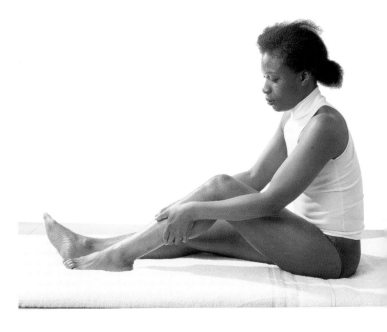

Shoulders and Neck

This is a good way to release tension and also help to reduce a headache. Begin in a sitting position with your back held straight. Take your hands up to your neck and from the base to the hairline use firm stroking or gliding movements one after the other. Create circular pressure movements with the tips of your fingers on either side of your spine up your neck and around your hairline. You can adjust the firmness accordingly.

Move your cupped hands up and down your calves to relieve aches and pains effectively.

Lower Arms

Either as part of a hand massage or separately, use upward strokes from wrist to elbow, adjusting firmness as necessary. Hold your arm between your fingers to apply pressure to aches.

Relieve tension in your neck and shoulders by squeezing the muscles gently between your fingers and the heel of your hand, applying pressure with your fingertips.

Legs

A leg massage can soothe aches and pains caused by standing too long or act as a pain reliever for overexercised muscles. Sit on your bed or floor with one knee up and use both hands to cup your leg. Stroke the whole leg from ankle to thigh by moving your cupped hands up and along. Using the pummel movement, pummel the tops and outsides of your thighs to help to bring blood to the surface and relieve any stiffness. Use the kneading movement to ease tension from the calves, and finish by using stroking movements from ankle to knee, one after the other.

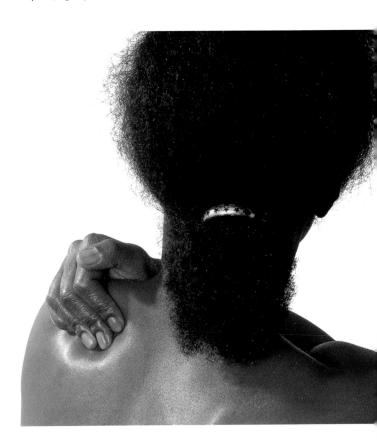

Tip 95: *Good Posture*

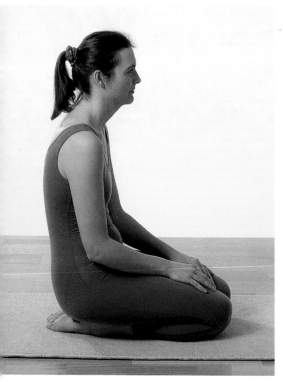

1. Slouching is depleting: back muscles are affected, breathing is impaired and the functioning of digestion and the abdominal organs is impeded.

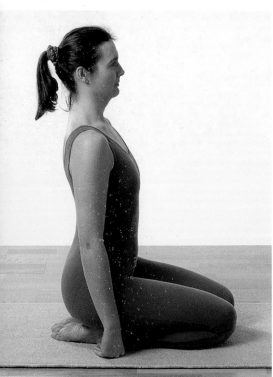

2. Sitting with a thrust-out chest also affects back muscles. It can easily impede the nervous system and results in shallow and ineffectual breathing.

Posture, or the way you sit and stand, has a huge impact on keeping the body – in particular, the spine – healthy. At one time or another, most of us have experienced back pain, and maintaining good posture is vital to reducing the likelihood of it coming back. Not only does having poor posture strain muscles and put stress on the spine, but it can also constrict the blood vessels causing poor blood flow, leading to headaches, tiredness and even breathing incorrectly. Good posture means having each part of the body in alignment with other parts, and movements such as sitting, standing, bending or lying down should be fluid and smooth, with no jarring or groan-inducing movements! It is possible to learn correct movements that lead to good posture, and these are a low-maintenance way of keeping the body pain-free. Specific everyday culprits that are likely to cause back pain include slouching (shoulders forward rather than back), holding a phone under your chin resting on your shoulder, carrying a heavy bag on one side, wearing high heels or sleeping on a mattress that doesn't give proper support to the spine. Office workers are often at risk of back pain due to poor posture. It is essential not to slump at your desk (relaxing the spine so the back is curved) and to take breaks from a sitting position as often as possible. Identifying your own posture problems can be done by being aware of aches and twinges and making a note of when they occur. Noting which positions cause discomfort and pain during the day can reveal the problem and let you solve it. There are many followers of the Alexander Technique, which uses a method of changing positional habits so that movements become free and support balance and co-ordination. Although the Alexander Technique should be taught by a qualified teacher, there are a couple of simple exercises that anyone can try. First, using a small pile of books about

2 inches (5 cm) high to rest your head on, lie on the floor with your knees bent upward, spine flat to the floor, with your head resting on your books. Do this for 15 minutes to give your spine a thorough stretch.

It is also believed that the way you breathe can have an impact on your body's ability to function properly. An easy technique to try is to sit in a chair and make yourself comfortable. Be aware of how you are sitting. Are you slouching or sitting upright? Now stand as you normally would and register how you stood up – you may have needed to place your hands on the arms of the chair to give yourself the lift. Try it again, using Alexander principles. This time, sit upright in your chair with your head relaxing slightly upward. Imagine a line traveling through the top of your head and down your spine. Stand up, keeping the line straight without using anything to force yourself upward and don't push with your knees. Simply lean forward and direct your body upward. You will notice that no pushing is necessary and this way of standing up places far less tension on your back or neck.

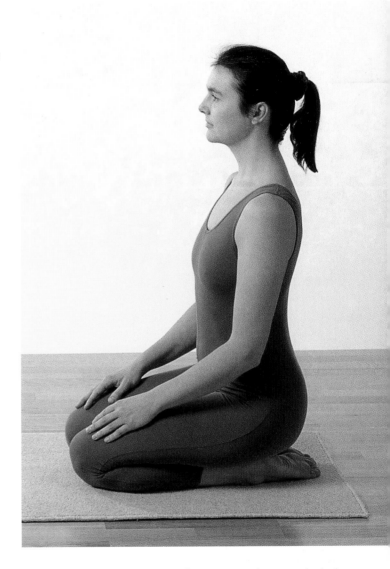

3. The need for an upright, but not rigid posture cannot be overemphasized. These pictures are posed is a simple seating position, but chairs, sensibly used, are just as effective. Sitting well, you are both more mentally alert and are using your body in a healthy way.

Tip 96: *Aromatherapy*

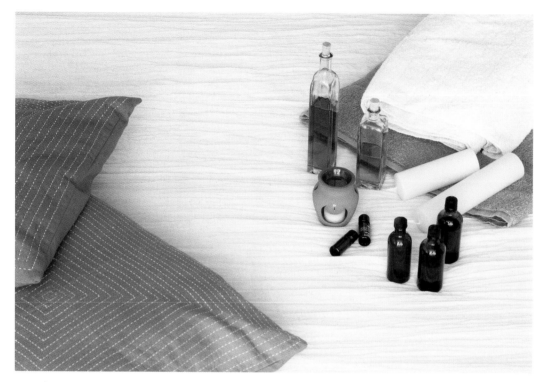

Essential oils can be used in massage to treat specific ailments or just to help you relax and unwind.

Aromatherapy is reputed to be at least 6,000 years old, and is believed to have been practiced by most of the world's ancient civilizations. Early humans lived closely with their surroundings and were in tune with nature. Their sense of smell was highly acute and herbs and aromatics were commonly used in the preservation of food, as digestive aids or to treat a variety of ailments. Aromatherapy means "treatment using scents" and is a holistic way of treating many symptoms, including stress. It can also be used in skin care, to alleviate tiredness and to treat pain. Using the sense of smell as a way of stimulating the nervous system and brain, aromatherapy is a popular and increasingly common holistic therapy. Essential oils can be intensely stimulating and the sense of smell a powerful one, thought to reach the part of the brain that controls mood, memory and emotions. Different smells can trigger different responses, and there are over 150 essential oils used in the practice of aromatherapy, each one either in combination or alone to target specific problems.

A full aromatherapy treatment is a truly wonderful experience, combining, as it does, the beneficial properties of the essential oils with the warm relaxing atmosphere of a well-prepared massage and possibly the enjoyment of some soothing music. As a holistic form of treatment, aromatherapy aims to deal with the underlying cause of the complaint, as well as the symptoms, and the form of treatment is very important when dealing with stress-related problems as a physical symptom is more often than not a manifestation of an underlying psychological or emotional problem. You may want to visit an aromatherapy practitioner to find out whether these treatments are for you, but there are several aromatherapy practices that you can use at home for day-to-day relaxation.

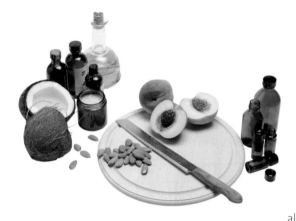

A popular way to use the therapeutic benefits of aromatherapy is through massage. Depending upon what mood you want to create, aromatherapy massage can be stimulating, sensual or relaxing. Oils are absorbed into the skin and inhaled while the massage takes place. You can use this method to self-massage or have someone else massage you. The benefits of aromatherapy massage are that it also eases muscle tension or aches and pains. By adding several drops of essential oil to the bath, you create a haven of relaxation, and the oils are absorbed via the skin and through inhaling the natural steam from your bath water. Inhaling essential oils can be done by adding three or four drops of your chosen oil to a bowl of steaming warm water and placing a towel over your head and the bowl to channel the vapors. This treatment is useful for those who suffer from headaches, sinus problems or who simply want an intense relaxation experience. Using a diffuser or burner can give an entire room a different feel by choosing either an invigorating, comforting or sensual oil. It can also help to aid concentration or be used to freshen the air. Aromatherapy compresses are often used to alleviate headaches or aches and pains. Massage the area that is painful with your oil and then cover with a hot or cold washcloth. It is important to remember that aromatherapy oils should never be used on their own, but always in a carrier oil, such as wheatgerm, avocado or sweet almond. It is always advisable to check labeling or consult an aromatherapist during pregnancy as some oils are deemed unsuitable for use at this time.

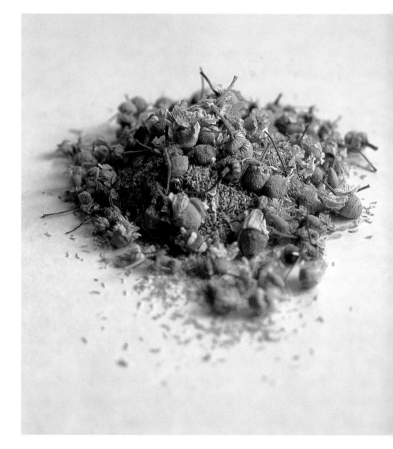

Aromatherapy oils are made from natural ingredients such as plants and herbs. They are crushed to extract their healing properties.

Tip 97: *Reflexology*

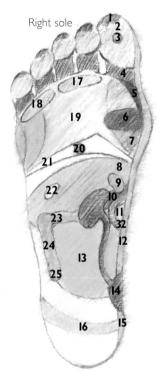
Right sole

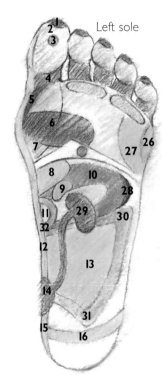
Left sole

1. Brain. 2. Head and sinus. 3. Pituitary gland. 4. Thyroid, neck and parathyroid. 5. Thymus. 6. Heart. 7. Thyroid area. 8. Liver. 9. Adrenal glands. 10. Stomach. 11. Pancreas. 12. Spinal region. 13. Small intestine. 14. Bladder. 15. Tailbone area. 16. Sciatic nerve. 17. Eyes. 18. Ears. 19. Lungs. 20. Solar plexus. 21. Diaphragm. 22. Gallbladder. 23. Transverse colon. 24. Ascending colon. 25. Ileocal valve. 26. Arms. 27. Shoulders. 28. Spleen. 29. Kidney. 30. Descending colon. 31. Sigmoid colon. 32. Duodenum.

This ancient Chinese technique uses pressure point massage, most commonly on the feet, to restore the flow of energy throughout the body. It is a complementary therapy that uses a principle of "whole body" healing via the feet and hands, and uses a mix of stretching, movement and pressure. It is thought that areas on the feet or hands directly link to other body parts via the nervous system, and that by applying pressure to these links, sensory nerves carry information to the brain, in turn stimulating it to function in another body part more effectively. The benefits of reflexology are thought to be mainly related to stress reduction and restoration of equilibrium. After a long day, it is a natural reaction to kick off your shoes and rub your feet – an instinctive action that mimics reflexology, so you may have done some basic reflexology without realizing it! To try some home reflexology, it is best to use either your computer to download a reflexology chart or to buy a chart available at any good health or complementary therapy store. The chart outlines which parts of the feet relate to other

organs. Reflexology is easily done in the bath or while relaxing in a comfortable chair. Aim to ensure your feet are washed first, and do not massage any areas that are tender, cut, inflamed or bruised. Using an oil or lotion, your hands can flow easily over your feet, but take care when standing up as your feet may still be slippery. After locating the areas you want to target, use fingers, knuckles or palms to massage. You should not be in any discomfort but exert a reasonable amount of pressure. A very simple way to enjoy the benefits of reflexology without the aid of chart is to invest in a foot tub that will produce bubbles and jets to gently give your feet an all-over treatment.

Some practitioners believe that treatment should not be attempted during pregnancy or if you have heart problems, thrombosis or shingles. If in any doubt, ask your doctor.

A good technique is the thumb/caterpillar walking technique, which is on the opposite page.

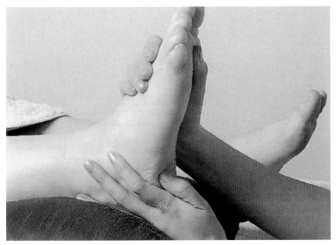

1. To walk the thumb, bend only the first joint of the thumb slightly and then unbend the joint slightly. The walking movement is always performed forward, never backward.

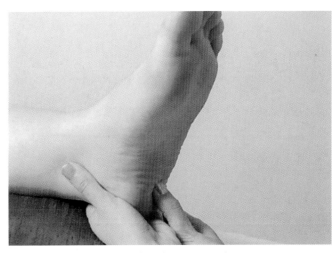

2. Move to a different part of the foot, ensuring that you maintain a constant, steady and even pressure.

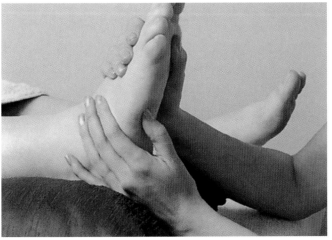

3. An on-off-on-off pressure should not be felt at each bend of the thumb. Do not worry if your thumbs start to ache or feel sore at first. Make sure you cover the edges of the foot, too.

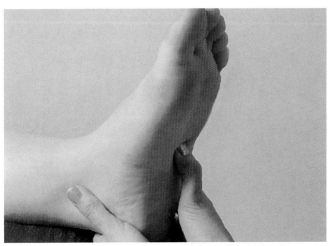

4. When carrying out this technique toward the bottom of the foot, ensure you get leverage by cupping the heel with your four fingers.

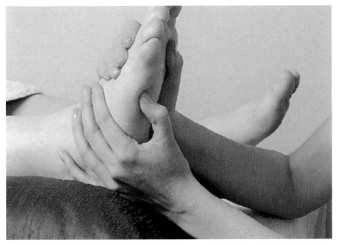

5. As the thumb is walking, the four fingers should be molded to the contours of the foot.

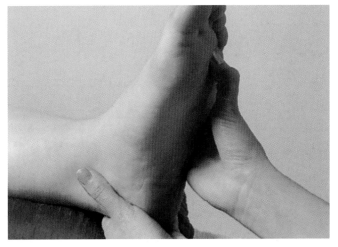

6. The four fingers should be kept together comfortably to ensure maximum leverage. If they are spread out then some of the leverage will be lost.

Tip **98**: *Meditation*

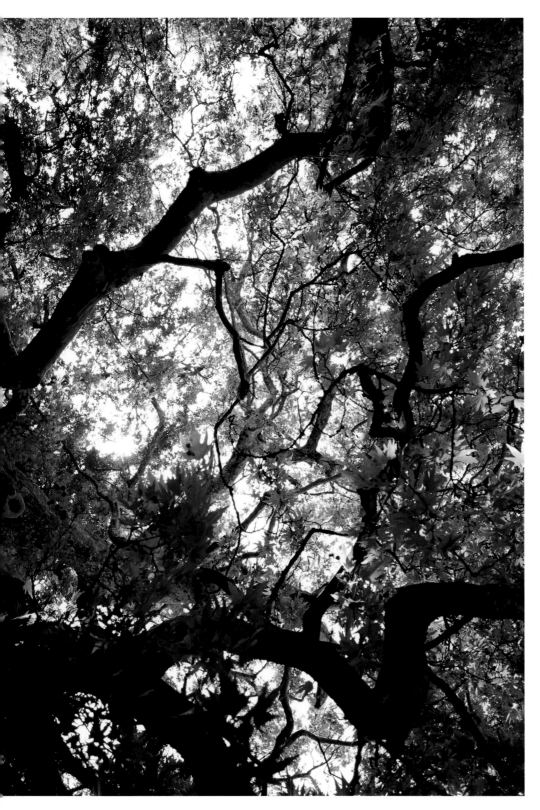

Used commonly as a relaxation technique, meditation in its varying forms is the practice of focusing the mind. It is used in religious practices, complementary therapies and spirituality, with different traditions and different treatments using a variety of techniques and physical positions. However, although extremely varied in approach, the fundamentals of meditation are accessible to everyone. Try these basic meditation techniques at home to enjoy a few moments of stillness and calm. Ensure that the room you use to meditate in is free of noise and distractions, is warm and comfortable and that you won't be disturbed. It can be a good idea to focus on something relaxing and calming in your mind. This will help you to forget about your daily worries and make you more able to relax.

Relaxation is commonly associated with having nothing on our mind that we feel we need to do. We say we relax in front of the television, in the backyard or in the local coffee shop. These forms of relaxation certainly are a welcome break from the daily grind. But while doing these things, our spine might be twisted, hips turned awkwardly or arms and legs under pressure from each other. Our mind might start wandering, turning over worries and concerns, or simply daydreaming. We might be drinking alcohol, taking stimulants or eating junk food. Relaxation through meditation is different. In meditation we turn our attention to our whole being, using the power of our mind to relax our whole being. Breathing and movement are crucial elements of meditation, particularly breathing. A lot of meditation is carried out still, but slow deliberate movements can be used very effectively to focus the mind.

Basic Meditation Technique Using Breathing

Lie comfortably on a blanket or rug on the floor or on a bed and enjoy the stillness for a few seconds, trying to let your thoughts calm. Allow your breathing to become deep and regular and focus on the weight of your body on the floor. In your mind, name your body parts, beginning at your toes and working all the way through to the head, focusing on any areas of tension you feel. For a count of five, allow your body to tense, inhale a deep breath, and relax your body while pushing out the air you have just taken in. By focusing on your breathing you may find that it is easier to clear your mind of other thoughts. Breathing in through the nose and out through the mouth, ensure you take deep breaths, holding the air inside your lungs for a

couple of seconds before you exhale. Keep focusing on your breathing; if your mind starts to wander, don't worry, just refocus on the breath sounds and get back in rhythm. Give yourself several minutes and then bring your attention back to where you are.

Basic Meditation Technique Using Movement

Ensuring that you have sufficient space to move around freely, stand with your palms by your waist, closing your eyes and allow your body to move in whatever way feels natural. The movements should be slow and simple. Concentrate on keeping every part of the body loose, but don't overthink what you are doing. Allowing natural and free movements is how this exercise works best. You may find that moving one part of your body at a time works best to begin with. Try to sense your muscles moving, and focus in on areas that feel better for movement. To end this exercise, concentrate on your arms and hands, with your palms facing upward. Allow them to move freely for a moment or two thinking only about the movements you are making, and end the exercise by shaking out your limbs.

Left: Focusing on a relaxing scene such as a forest or a favorite landscape can heighten the relaxing effects of meditation.

Tip 99: *Essential Oils*

Essential oils are taken from plants, trees, fruits and seeds. Synthetic oils will not have the therapeutic effects that naturally extracted oils have. Most oils are generally suitable for home use. Essential oils have many uses, but those listed below are some of the most popular for treating stress and aiding relaxation. Remember to follow labels regarding dilution instructions and never apply pure essential oils to the skin.

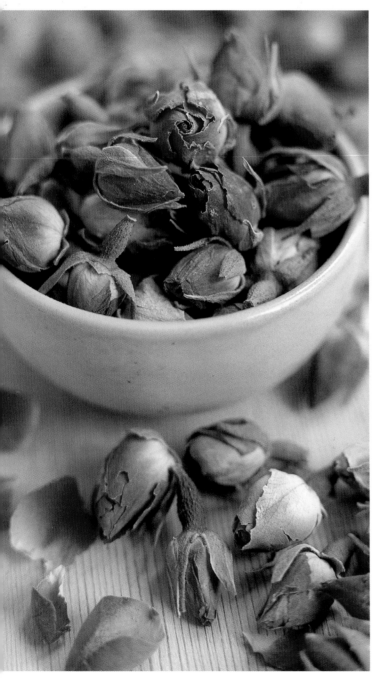

Geranium

With a multitude of relaxing properties, geranium is an excellent oil for soothing, relaxing, mood lifting and treating nervous tension. It is also thought to treat menopausal symptoms and act as a mild antidepressant, and it contains antiseptic properties.

Sage

This oil has warming and soothing properties, and is also thought to be an aphrodisiac! It too has antidepressive and antiseptic qualities and can be used in skin care to reduce wrinkles, act astringently on oily areas and calm inflamed patches. Practitioners also use sage to tackle throat infections, colic and migraine headaches.

Chamomile

This is traditionally used as a relaxant and antidepressant. It has been used to reduce preoperative anxiety, and also to help relieve the mood swings associated with premenstrual syndrome (PMS).

Rose

Oil from rose (pictured left) is traditionally considered useful for gynecological and women's hormonal problems, and the mood states that tend to accompany them. It is also used in skin care preparations for its ability to soften and restore youthful qualities to the skin and helping to reduce the redness of capillaries.

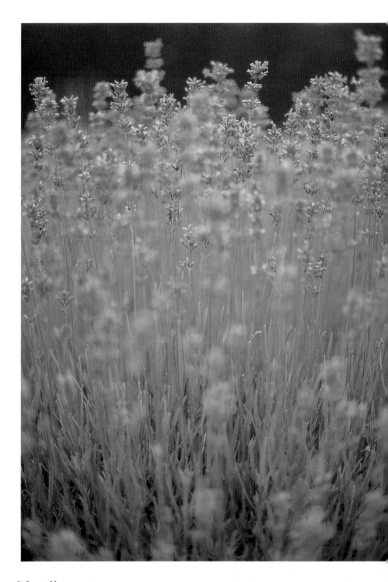

Jasmine

Jasmine is a very common oil for its benefits in raising the spirits. Thought to promote optimism and confidence and relieve stress, it can also treat skin problems such as dry and irritated areas.

Lavender

Probably one of the best known oils, lavender (pictured right) is reputed to have strong relaxation properties and is commonly used to aid sleep and reduce stress. Practitioners claim that it can help to alleviate depression, headaches, PMS and athlete's foot, and it is also a natural insect repellent.

Lemon

Citrus-based oils are naturally refreshing and uplifting, and often used to re-energize, stimulate and invigorate. Lemon oil has a wonderful, fresh fragrance and is a natural antiseptic.

Petitgrain

From the citrus family, this fragrance is soothing and calming and a natural mood enhancer, or pick-me-up. It can also help with skin disorders such as acne, overly oily skin and hair, and to tone.

Sandalwood

This is commonly thought to have beneficial effects on dry, cracked or chapped skin, and can be used to moisturize. The scent can relieve tension, ease stress and act as aphrodisiac.

Vanilla

Some sources suggest the use of vanilla as a remedy for anger, tension and irritability; others confirm the traditional use of vanilla as an aphrodisiac.

Ylang Ylang

This sweet smelling oil has several useful properties, including mood lifting, relaxing and treating insomnia. It is also thought to be an aphrodisiac and has abilities to stimulate the circulatory and nervous systems.

Tip 100: *Mud Therapies*

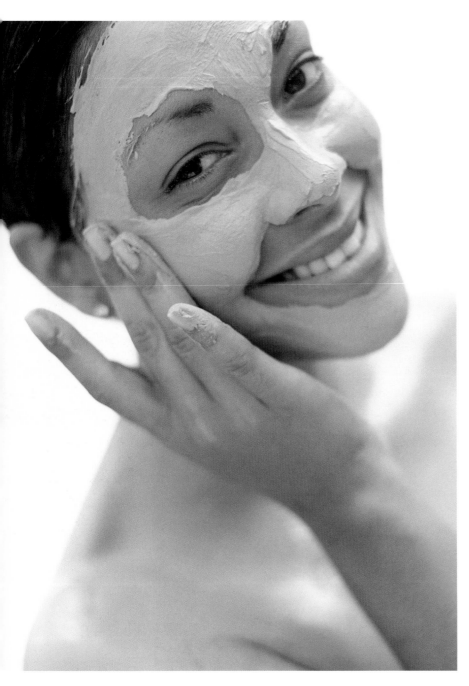

Mud face masks, which are often made from clay, are very effective at removing blackheads and other debris from the skin.

While it may not seem like the most tantalizing of treatments, the therapeutic uses of mud are centuries-old. Mud has the ability of being able to absorb, dissolve and eliminate toxins and has great benefits to the skin. In fact, in animal life, a mud wallow is a perfectly natural and highly efficient way to clean the skin! Muds work by transferring heat, which in turn accelerates the natural detoxification process. Several types of mineral-rich mud are commonly used in treatments, and these include moor muds, which are peat-based, fango, which is found in hot springs, clay, and brine muds, which come from coastal areas and contain high levels of salt. Mud treatments are also thought to help with conditions like rheumatism and joint swelling. While it is possible to buy mud packs for home use, the practicalities of an at-home mud bath are tricky. Mud, obviously, is loose in consistency and the process can be very messy. Finding somewhere to lie while your mud works its magic is always going to result in a sticky pile of laundry! However, mud face masks – usually clay-based – are easier to deal with and have great drawing properties to remove blackheads and debris. They tend to be more suitable for oily skin. Mud therapies can be applied in several ways. Commonly used in spas, a mud wrap treatment will consist of an initial exfoliation and then the application of (usually) warmed mud that is painted over the body. You are then wrapped in either cling film or bandaging, allowing the mud to absorb while its cleansing, toning and anti-inflammatory

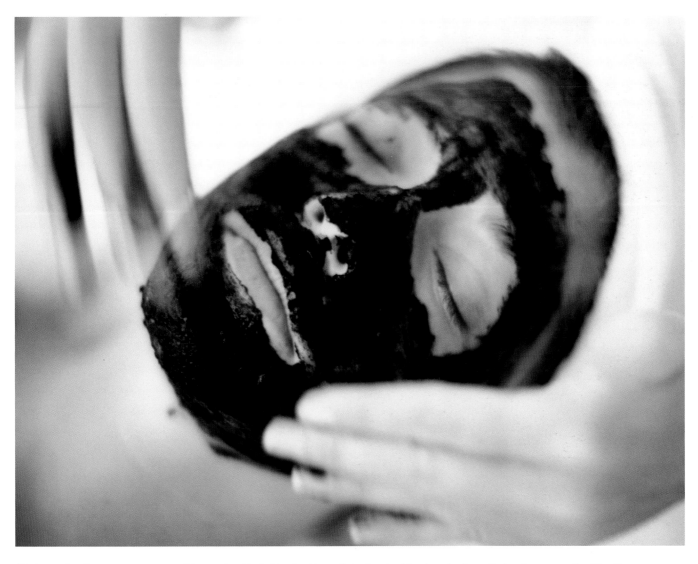

Mud is perfect for removing toxins and leaves the skin looking healthy and glowing. Applying it to the face will give the most noticeable effects, but all-over body treatments are available. These are very hard to apply successfully and cleanly at home, so try them at your local beauty salon.

properties get to work. Mud baths are less common, but are exactly what they sound like: a bath full of mud, or a combination of marine extracts and mud that you lie in for a period of time. A practice that originated in Arabic countries and is gaining in popularity is a "Rasul." This consists of several types of mud that are smoothed over the body. Using a sauna principle, a small, tiled room is then filled with steam, helping the therapeutic mud to work more deeply. After the steam comes a stream of water – or a shower – in which you can thoroughly cleanse away any last traces of mud.

Tip 101: *Sleeping Tips*

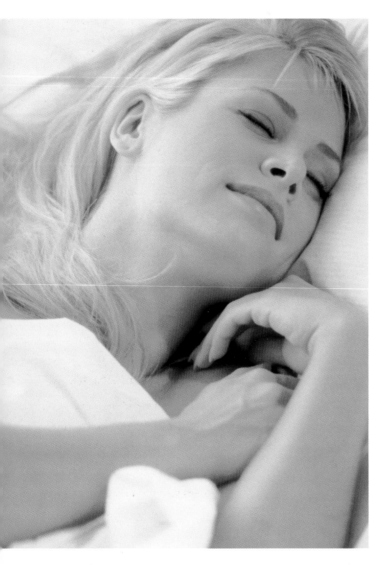

A good way to encourage sleep is to lie down and take deep, concentrated breaths. Breathe from within your abdomen to a count of three, then breathe out slowly to a count of three. Try this for around 10 minutes, and if it doesn't work, leave the bedroom and do something else.

Sleep is perhaps the most mysterious of all our natural body functions. Some of us sleep heavily, some of us sleep lightly and some of us hardly sleep at all. Patterns of sleep are almost as individual as the world's population itself, but we all know that not getting enough sleep is the cause of tiredness, misery and a general feeling of malaise. We know that that sleep waves and dreaming (or REM) phases occur, but there is little real knowledge of why, and what their importance might be. Even the experts agree that sleep studies are in their infancy. We can measure the effects of lack of sleep more easily than its benefits and make deductions from that, but fundamentally all we know is that the best cure for sleepiness is sleep itself. So what can be done to improve our chances of getting a good night's sleep?

Take breaths from deep within your abdomen (not the top of your chest), to a count of three. Breathe out slowly to a count of three. Try doing this over and over again for 10 minutes. If you still don't feel sleepy, move out of your bedroom and find something quiet to do. When you start to feel sleepy, go back to bed and try again. Sometimes something as simple as the condition of your bedroom can be the cause. Is your room unduly messy and stressful to be in? Is there a TV in the room? Keeping your room tidy sometimes help to keep the mind tidy too, and not assessing your room for things that need to be done can be relaxing in itself. Keep the TV out of the bedroom to avoid the temptation to switch it on and overstimulate your brain. Ensure you have low lighting and the room is at a comfortable temperature. Some people find that a few drops of lavender oil on their pillow can help. Ensure that you are active enough during the day; make a daily exercise routine a priority, but don't exercise too closely to bedtime. Despite popular belief, alcohol won't help you to sleep. While it is okay to have a small nightcap, too much alcohol will make you restless, and because it is a diuretic, you are more likely to need to visit the bathroom during the night. Alcohol can also cause snoring, restricting airflow and

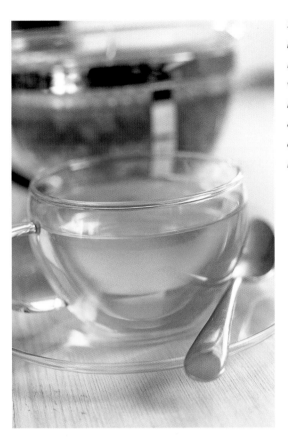

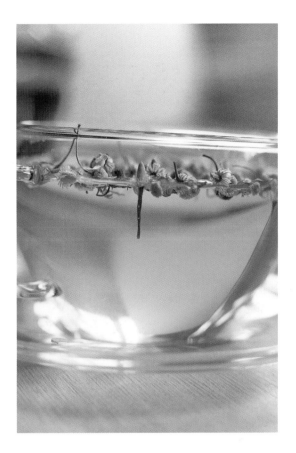

Some herbal teas have been shown to aid relaxation and help with sleep. Ensure that it is an herbal tea you are drinking, as ordinary tea contains caffeine and will inhibit sleep.

disturbing your rest. The same can be said of caffeine – there is nothing more guaranteed to ensure you need to make a middle of the night trip to the bathroom than a cup of tea or coffee, or a glass of cola. Stick to hot milk or herbal teas. Avoid eating too late at night as this can also play havoc with your sleep. Heartburn from fatty or very spicy foods can cause discomfort right through the night. You are far better to have a late snack that consists of carbohydrates, which are more likely to trigger the sleep-inducing hormone serotonin. Although it is thought to be an urban myth, the rumor that cheese gives you bad dreams is in part based on truth. Cheese (and other foods such as red wine, bacon and avocados) contains a substance called tyramine, which causes overstimulation. While eight hours is the average optimum amount of sleep, everyone is different. If you feel energetic, happy and well on four or five hours of sleep a night, there is no need to try to get more. It could be that this is just your natural requirement. It is thought by experts that just four hours of sleep a night equips the brain with most of the sleep benefits. Lastly, try not to nap in the daytime, however tired you feel. Napping that lasts longer than about 15 minutes can often have the effect of making us feel worse than we did to start with. Leave sleep to the bedroom. Try to get into a regular sleeping pattern. Getting up early is likely to help you to get to sleep early.

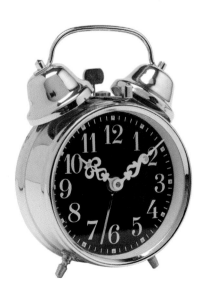

Ensure you get up at a reasonable hour and set your alarm if necessary. Do not be tempted to turn off your alarm and go back to sleep. Getting up early will help you to go to sleep early.

GLOSSARY

Acne – Spots caused by the overactivity of the *sebaceous glands* that secrete oily substances onto the skin.

Additives – any substance used in the production, processing, treatment, packaging, tranportation or storage of food. Most of the time, "additives" refers to the chemicals used to preserve, add flavor to or give color to food.

Aerobic exercise – activity which increases the heart rate and your intake of oxygen.

Alexander Technique – set of exercises designed to promote good posture.

Alpha Hydroxy Acids (AHAs) – ingredient found in some *moisturizers* and *antioxidant* night creams that helps to encourage cell renewal.

Anaerobic exercise – high intensity, short bursts of exercise such as weight lifting, press-ups and stomach crunches.

Anti-dandruff shampoos and conditioners – products containing selenium sulphide or zinc oxide that help to control the levels of *dandruff* produced on the scalp. Severe *dandruff* is treated with *shampoos* containing ketoconasole, an anti-fungal agent.

Antioxidants – substance found in foods such as plums, artichokes, blueberries and pomegranates that combat molecules called *free radicals*, which damage cells.

Aromatherapy – treatment of physical and emotional ailments using *essential oils*.

Aspartame – artifical sweetener added to some foods, which some scientists have linked with neurological damage.

B vitamins – vital for the health of the nervous system and to help release energy from the food we eat.

Balanced diet – diet that takes into account all the food groups, but with higher consumption of grains, fruits and vegetables than meats, dairy products and fats.

Blackheads – Caused by overactive *sebaceous glands*. When the glands produce too much *sebum* the pores of your skin become stretched and clogged. The *sebum* forms a hard plug and because the pore is open, the oil oxidizes, turning black.

Blending color – technique of applying makeup so that it looks seamless with no obvious stops and starts in color.

Blow-dryer – an electronic device that generates hot air to dry hair. Overuse can damage hair.

Blush – used to give color to the cheeks.

Blush brush – used to apply *blush* to the cheeks.

Body Mass Index (BMI) – height and weight calculation to discern whether you are underweight, overweight, obese or normal.

Botox – a highly diluted and purified form of the nerve toxin which causes botulism, a serious (and sometimes fatal) paralytic illness. Injected in tiny and safe quantities, it reduces the appearance of wrinkles.

Butylparaben – a chemical used in *makeup* and some skincare products to prolong shelf life. See also *Propylparaben* and *Parabens*.

Caffeine – Chemical found in coffee, some teas and soft drinks that can hamper the absorption of certain minerals into the body and can also affect your ability to fall asleep.

Calcium – mineral found in dairy products that is essential to healthy bones and teeth.

Carbohydrate – sugars and starches found in food that provide the body with energy.

Cationic surfactants – active ingredients used in commercial *conditioners* that are attracted to dry and damaged hair.

Cellulite – deposits of fat underneath the skin, which can give a dimpled "orange peel" appearance to the skin.

Chamomile – *essential oil* used as a relaxant and antidepressant.

Clary sage – *essential oil* with warming and soothing properties that is used to tackle depression, throat infections, colic and migraine.

Close-set eyes – eyes that look close together, with less than the usual space between them.

Collagen – ingredient added to some *moisturizers* that helps to disguise the appearance of wrinkles.

Combination skin – oily skin around the nose and across the forehead and chin, but normal or slightly *dry skin* elsewhere.

Comfrey – herb that is used to treat *acne*.

Concealers – used to disguise imperfections and blemishes on the skin.

Conditioner – product designed to leave hair smooth, tangle free and shiny.

Cool down – the gradual slowing down at the end of an exercise session to allow the heart and breathing rates to return to normal steadily.

Curling iron – electronic device used to style curls into the hair.

Dandruff – old discarded skin cells from the scalp. Everybody loses skin from the scalp as part of the natural process of skin renewal, but this process happens quicker on people with dandruff.

Deep-set eyes – eyes that look set much deeper than the cheek bones.

Dehydration – lack of fluids in the body leading to thirst, lightheadedness and impaired muscle performance.

Depilatory creams – remove unwanted hair from just below the surface of the skin using chemicals.

Detangling spray – a product designed to help detangle hair.

Dry hair – hair without enough moisture. It lacks shine, tangles easily and feels rough.

Dry skin – skin that is lacking in natural oils and is prone to aging.

Effleurage – basic massage stroke.

Electrolysis – a method of removing unwanted hair by passing a small amount of energy via a fine needle through the hair follicle. This produces heat that destroys the root.

Endorphins – "feel good" hormones released into the brain during exercise.

Epilators – Electrical tweezing heads that rotate over the skin, removing hair as they go

Essential fats – "good" fats such as *monounsaturated* and essential fatty acids such as *Omega 3* and 6.

Essential oils – oils derived from plants, trees, fruits and seeds used in *aromatherapy* to treat physical and emotional ailments.

Exfoliating – the process of removing dead skin cells with abrasive tools or creams.

Exfoliating gels and creams – cleansers that contain tiny natural grains or man-made spheres to exfoliate the skin.

Eye shadow brush – blunt-tipped brush used to apply *eyeshadow*.

Eyedrops – used to give the eyes added sparkle.

Eyelash curlers – tool used to create beautifully upturned lashes.

Eyeliner – added to define the eyes.

Eyeshadow – used to add color to the eyelids, available as powder or creams.

Face masks – treatment used to remove impurities from the skin.

False eyelashes – can be worn to give the effect of longer, fuller eyelashes.

Fiber – essential for a healthy lifestyle, it promotes good digestion and can lower blood cholesterol and may even reduce bowel cancer. There are two types of fiber – *soluble* and *insoluble*.

Flat paddle brush – a brush designed for flat hair.

Flaxseed oil – an oil that is high in *Omega-3 fatty acids*.

Folic acid – a *B vitamin* that plays a key role in the health and development of cells. Women who are trying to become pregnant should ensure that their diet is rich in folic acid, as it helps to aid the healthy development of fetuses.

Foundation – used to even out skin tones, giving the complexion a healthy, "flawless" look. Available in different colors and textures.

Free radicals – molecules found in the body that can damage cells.

Friction – basic massage stroke.

Geranium – *essential oil* used for soothing, relaxing, mood lifting, treating nervous tension, treating menopausal symptoms and as a mild antidepressant.

GI (glycemic index) diet – Foods classified into low, medium or high GI depending on the rate they release energy into the body. The diet emphasizes the importance of low-GI foods, which release energy slower and therefore sustain you for longer.

Hair breakage – damage to the hair caused by *perming, relaxing treatments, hair extensions* and bleaching. Can also be caused by a medical condition.

Hair cuticles – the outer hair cells.

Hair dyes – products used to change the color of the hair.

Hair extensions – made from either human hair or synthetic fibers, hair extensions bond to your own hair to add length and increase the scope for styling.

Heart face – characterized by a wide forehead with the face narrowing toward the chin.

Heat protection spray – a product designed to stop the hair drying out and to prevent heat related damage, such as *split ends* and frizz. Essential if you regularly blow dry your hair.

Highlighter – used to brighten and enhance your face, and to give emphasis to your best features. Available as highlighter pencils or cream highlighter.

Humectant – a technical word used to describe a hair product that draws moisture to the hair. Products that use the word "moisturizing" will have the same effect.

Hydrolipidic film – the naturally occurring thin, oily layer on the surface of the skin.

Insoluble fiber – found in wholewheat cereals, rice and many fruit and vegetables, it is essential for healthy bowel funtion and may even ward against bowel cancer.

Ionic brush – a brush generates negative ions to smooth the hair shaft, which helps to combat static and flyaway hair.

Jasmine – *essential oil* used to relieve stress and promote well-being.

Keratin – the protein that hair is made of.

Kneading – basic massage technique.

Lactic acid – a chemical compound that plays a role in fueling the cells, but is more commonly used as a phrase to describe the tired feeling and soreness in the muscles brought on by intensive exercise.

Lanolin – greasy substance from wool-bearing animals, which is used in some *dry skin* and dry lip treatments.

Laser hair removal – high intensity light providing heat energy is used to damage or destroy the hair roots. Not effective for people with gray, white, blond or light red hair, as the laser targets the pigment.

Lavender – *essential oil* used as a relaxant, to aid sleep and reduce stress.

Lemon – *essential oil* used for its uplifting and invigorating properties.

Limbic area – the part of the brain responsible for the emotions. Practitioners of *aromatherapy* believe that *essential oils* act upon this area of the brain.

Lip balm – used to treat chapped lips, but also smooth eyebrows and to give a sheen effect to the cheeks.

Lip brush – used to give more accurate application of color than a *lipstick*.

Lip gloss – adds color and shine to the lips.

Lip pencil – used to give outline to the lips.

Lipstick – adds color to the lips, with a more matte effect than *lip gloss*.

Long face – characterized by long and angular features, with most of the length being from the eye to the chin area.

Loofah – natural exfoliant made from dried dishcloth gourd (luffa), a soft, fibrous plant.

Low-density lipoprotein (LDL) – harmful cholesterol produced by the overconsumption of *saturated fats*.

Magnesium – plays a role in the production and transport of energy. It is also important for the contraction and relaxation of muscles. Magnesium is involved in the synthesis of *protein*, and it assists in the functioning of certain enzymes in the body. A lack of magnesium can lead to dry and brittle hair.

Mascara – added to emphasize eyelashes, available as a block or as a liquid wand.

Meditation – technique of focused relaxation thought to promote wellbeing and to combat stress.

Moisturizers – products used to hydrate the skin, making it softer and more flexible.

Monosodium glutamate – food additive that has been linked to nerve cell damage and cancer.

Monounsaturated fats – healthy fat when consumed at recommended levels. Found in olive oil, canola (rapeseed) oil, nuts and avocado.

Mud therapies – application of special mud to the skin to eliminate toxins.

Narrow/small eyes – eyes that have a narrow, "squinting" appearance.

Normal skin – the ideal type of skin that is neither too dry nor too oily.

Nylon scrub – a machine-washable exfoliant.

Obesity – dangerous level of weight for a person's height and body type. It is linked with an increase risk of heart disease and *Type 2 diabetes*.

Oily hair – hair that is covered with *sebum*, the natural secretion of the *sebaceous glands* in the scalp. *Sebum* passes into the hair follicle and lies on the hair shafts.

Oily skin – skin that looks shiny and is prone to *blackheads*, linked to the overproduction of *sebum*.

Omega-3 fatty acids – An essential nutrient found in salmon, mackerel, tuna and other oily fish that has a number of health benefits, such as strengthening skin, nails and hair. Also linked to brain and visual development and health.

Omega-6 fatty acids – An essential nutrient found in meat and vegetable oils. Although essential, consumption in the developed world is too high and overconsumption is linked to illnesses such as heart disease.

Osteoporosis – disease that causes the bones to become weaker as women get older.

Oval face – characterized by a square chin, a wide, high forehead and flat sides.

Parabens – chemicals used in makeup and some skincare products to prolong shelf life, usually referred to as *Butylparaben* and *Propylparaben*.

Para-phenylenediamine – a chemical found in some *hair dyes* that has been linked to an increased risk of bladder cancer. See also *Tetrahydro-6-nitroquinoxaline*.

Percussion – group of basic massage strokes.

Perming – the process of adding very defined curls to the hair.

Petitgrain – *essential oil* that is used for its soothing and invigorating properties.

Petrissage – basic massage technique.

Phthalates – chemicals used in cosmetics to add flexibility and to give an oily, moisturizing film.

Pick or Afro comb – a brush designed for very curly hair or Afro-Caribbean hair.

Plucking – a method of removing hair using *tweezers*.

Polyunsaturated fats – healthier than *saturated fats* but without the benefits of *monounstaurated fats*. Found in sunflower oil, corn oils and some vegetables.

Powder – applied on top of *foundation* to give matte finish and to prevent the *foundation* from streaking or running.

Primers – substance for the skin that allows *foundation* to be applied with more fluidity.

Problem skin – skin that is prone to flare-ups of pimples, blemishes and *blackheads* that don't heal easily.

Propylparaben – a chemical used in makeup and some skincare products to prolong shelf life. See also *Butylparaben* and *Parabens*.

Protein – essential for healthy bones and muscles.

Pumice – small pieces of volcanic rock that can be used to remove dead skin from the soles of the feet.

Pure bristle brush – tool used for *exfoliating*.

Reflexology – treatment of ailments by stimulating areas on the soles of the feet.

Relaxed treatment – a chemical treatment for Afro-Caribbean hair that straightens out tight curls.

REM (Rapid Eye Movement) – phase of sleep when dreaming takes place.

Rose – *essential oil* used for skincare and for the treatment of women's hormonal problems.

Round barrel brush – a brush designed to style curls into the hair.

Round face – characterized by full cheeks, a symmetrical appearance and uniform size.

Saccharin – artificial sweetener banned in Canada and some other countries after being linked to digestive problems and even some cancers.

Sandalwood – essential oil used to treat dry or chapped skin, as well as to relieve tension and ease stress.

Saturated fats – most unhealthy fat that can lead to the build up of unhealthy levels of *LDL* cholesterol if overconsumed.

Sebaceous glands – glands on the skin that secrete *sebum*, an oil that in moderate levels is essential for keeping the skin hydrated.

Seborrheoic dermatitis – a condition of the scalp that causes severe *dandruff*. Can be treated with *shampoos* containing ketoconasole, an anti-fungal agent.

Sebum – the secretion of the *sebaceous glands* on the skin and the scalp. Too much sebum is linked to oily skin and hair.

Sensitive skin – skin that reacts to weather conditions and certain beauty products and makeup.

Shampoo – cleaning product for the hair.

Shaving – a method of removing unwanted hair.

Silicone-based serum – a product that can be used to aid the detangling of hair.

Sisal – a fibrous plant that is ideal for *exfoliating*.

Soluble fiber – found in foods such as oats, beans and barley, it is beleieved to have a role in lowering cholesterol.

Sparkling body gel – used to give the skin a sparkling effect and can also be added to the face, but not near the eyes.

Split ends – damage to the hair when the protective cuticle has been stripped away from the ends of hair fibers. Split ends are more likely to develop in dry or brittle hair, and typical causes of damage include excessive dying or clumsy brushing.

Sponge applicator – used to apply *foundation*.

Sponges – can be used to wash the skin and as a gentle exfoliant.

Straightening iron – electronic device used to straighten curly hair.

Stretch marks – Silvery lines on the surface of the skin resulting from stretching and the breakage of small connective fibers beneath the skin.

Styling mousse – product used to style hair. Overuse can damage hair.

Styling spray – product used to style hair. Overuse can damage hair.

Sudan 1 – food coloring linked to cancer that has been removed from food agency "safe lists" and is no longer added to food.

Sugaring – a technique for removing hair that is similar to *waxing*. A sugary paste is applied to the skin, then rolled away, uprooting the hairs as it is done so. See also *Waxing*.

Sulphur dioxide – common additive in soft drinks that has been linked to gastric problems.

Sun Protection Factor – number used to measure how effective a lotion is at protecting the skin from the sun.

Tetrahydro-6-nitroquinoxaline – a chemical found in some *hair dyes* that has been linked to an increased risk of bladder cancer. See also *Para-phenylenediamine*.

Threading – a method of removing unwanted hair. Threaders use lenths of lopped cotton to catch and pull out the hairs.

Tick lip pencil – used to add color to the lips.

Tide marks – demarcation lines between the face and neck caused by incorrectly colored *foundation*, or a base that hasn't been blended properly.

Tinted Moisturizer – *moisturizer* that adds color to the skin.

Trans fatty acids – created when a process of "hydrogenation" is applied to vegetable oils. Found in processed and fast foods, trans fatty acids are very unhealthy and should be avoided.

Trichologists – Experts in scalp and hair problems – the different types of hair loss, baldness, scaling problems that occur, and the non-medical treatment of those conditions.

Tweezers – tool used for *plucking* eyebrows.

Type 2 diabetes – condition where the body is unable to regulate the amount of glucose in the body properly. It is the type of diabetes most linked to diet and lifestyle, but is also linked to genetic factors. Unlike Type 1 diabetes, the pancreas does not stop making insulin, but insulin production can be lowered or the body can stop responding to it.

Tyramine – substance found in foods such as cheese, red wine, bacon and avocado that is thought to lead to disturbed sleep and bad dreams.

USDA food guide pyramid – set of dietary recommendations that translates the suggested number of servings of various sorts of foods into a graphic image.

UVA – rays from the sun that can lead to skin damage.

UVB – rays from the sun that are the main cause of sunburn and skin cancer.

Vanilla – *essential oil* used as a remedy for anger, tension and irritability.

Vitamin A – a nutrient linked to healthy skin, good eyesight and the body's ability to combat infections.

Vitamin B2 – nutrient that is essential for healthy cells and cell growth.

Vitamin C – important for the health of skin, hair and the immune system.

Vitamin D – aids mineral absorption and promotes good bone health.

Vitamin E – nutrient with *antioxidant* properties, which can be used on *dry skin* and lips. Some scientists believe it also lessens the risk of developing heart disease and possibly come cancers.

Vitamins B6 and B12 – found in fresh fruit and vegetables, these vitamins are particularly important for healthy hair.

Warm-up – gentle exercise and stretching that helps to prepare the body for more strenuous activity.

Waxing – one way of removing unwanted hair. Liquid wax can be applied to the skin then stripped away or you can use waxing strips, which are strengthened strips of paper coated with a sticky wax designed to cling to hair. See also *Sugaring*.

Wide-set eyes – eyes that look like they have more than the usual space between them.

Wide-toothed comb – specially designed comb for wet hair.

Wigs and hairpieces – can be placed on the scalp to give the impression of real hair.

Ylang ylang – *essential oil* used stimulate the circulatory and nervous systems and also for mood lifting, relaxing and insomnia.

Zinc – plays an important role in the proper functioning of the immune system in the body. It is required for the enzyme activities necessary for cell division, cell growth, and wound healing. It plays a role in the acuity of the senses of smell and taste. Zinc is also involved in the metabolism of *carbohydrates*. A lack of zinc can lead to dry and brittle hair.

INDEX